Diagnosis in color

Cardiology

Adam Timmis
MA, MD, FRCP, FESC

Stephen Brecker
MD, MRCP

Consultant Cardiologist
London Chest Hospital
London

Consultant Cardiologist
St George's Hospital
London

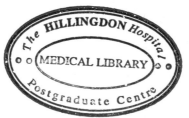

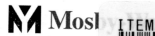

Mosby

London · Baltimore · Barcelona · Bogotá · Boston
· Madrid
lew York
ingapore
den

Project Manager:	**Leslie Sinoway**
Development Editors:	**Jennifer Prast**
	Gina Almond
Editorial Assisstant	**Nina Whitby**
Production:	**Gudrun Hughes**
Index:	**John Gibson**
Cover Design:	**Greg Smith**
Publisher:	**Claire Hooper**

Copyright © 1997 Times Mirror International Publishers Limited

Published in 1997 by Mosby-Wolfe, an imprint of Times Mirror International Publishers Limited

Printed in Italy by Vincenzo Bona s.r.l., Turin.

ISBN 0 7234 2551 5

Contents

1.

Introduction

1.1a–c   12 lead electrocardiogram

The electrocardiogram (ECG) records the electrical activity of the heart at the skin surface. It consists of three bipolar leads (I, II, III) and nine unipolar leads (aVR, aVL, aVF, V1–V6). The orientation of each lead with respect to the heart is different and, consequently, the positive and negative depolarization changes recorded by each lead are also different. However, the sequence of changes is always the same, each sinus impulse initiating atrial depolarization (P wave) followed by ventricular depolarization (QRS complex) and ventricular repolarization (T wave). The ECG is recorded at a paper speed of 25 mm/s such that each small square (1 mm) represents 0.04 s and each large square (5 mm) represents 0.20 s. The square wave is a calibration signal: 1 cm vertical deflection = 1 mV.

In analysing the ECG, the rate, rhythm and frontal plane QRS axis should be noted. Examination of P wave and QRS morphology provides evidence not only of myocardial disease involving the atria and ventricles but also conducting tissue disease as it affects the PR interval, the duration of the QRS complex and the association between the P wave and the QRS complex. ST segment analysis is important for the diagnosis of acute ischaemia, myocardial infarction and pericarditis.

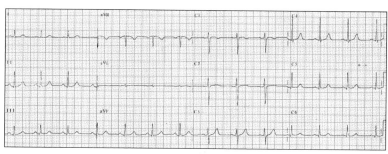

1.1a   Normal recording.

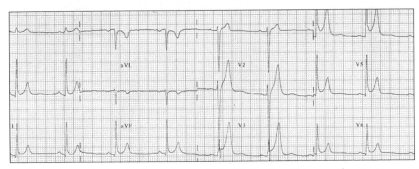

1.1b Early ventricular repolarization results in ST elevation. This normal variant is particularly common in people of Afro-Caribbean origin.

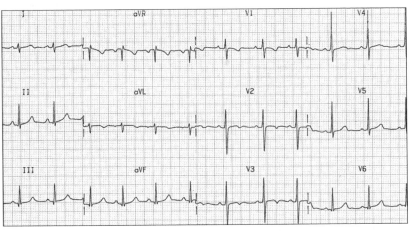

1.1c T wave inversion in leads V1–V3 is consistent with ischaemia in the anteroseptal territory but is commonly seen as a normal variant, particularly in women.

1.2 a and b   Sinus rhythm

The sinus node is the pacemaker of the normal heart. It depolarizes spontaneously at regular intervals which determines the heart rate. The sinus node is influenced by a variety of neurohumoral factors, particularly vagal and sympathetic activity which slow and quicken the heart rate, respectively. Each sinus discharge produces atrial depolarization (P wave) followed by ventricular depolarization (QRS complex) and ventricular repolarization (T wave). This sequence of ECG deflections occurring at regular intervals is the hallmark of sinus rhythm.

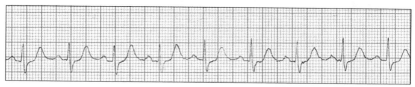

1.2a Normal sinus rhythm.

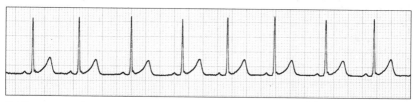

1.2b Sinus arrhythmia. In children and young adults the heart rate accelerates during inspiration and slows during expiration in response to phasic variations in sympathovagal balance.

Intervals		
The normal ECG intervals		
P wave	0.06–0.10 seconds	
PR interval	0.12–0.20 seconds	
QRS complex	0.08–0.10 seconds	
QT interval	0.35–0.42 seconds	

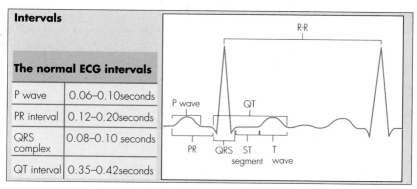

1.3 The normal ECG intervals

The PR interval represents the time taken for the sinus node impulse to reach the ventricular myocardium. Prolongation occurs when conduction through the AV node is delayed by disease or drugs (1° AV block). If AV conduction fails, either intermittently (2° AV block) or completely (3° AV block), the normal 1:1 relationship between P wave and QRS complex is lost. A short PR interval occurs when an accessory pathway bypasses the AV node permitting early ventricular activation (Wolff–Parkinson–White syndrome). It also occurs in low atrial or coronary sinus escape rhythms because of the proximity of the escape focus to the AV node.

The QT interval is very rate sensitive, shortening as the heart rate increases. Abnormal prolongation predisposes to ventricular arrhythmias and these may be congenital or occur in response to hypokalaemia, rheumatic fever or drugs (e.g. amiodarone, tricyclic antidepressants). Shortening of the QT interval is caused by hyperkalaemia and digoxin therapy.

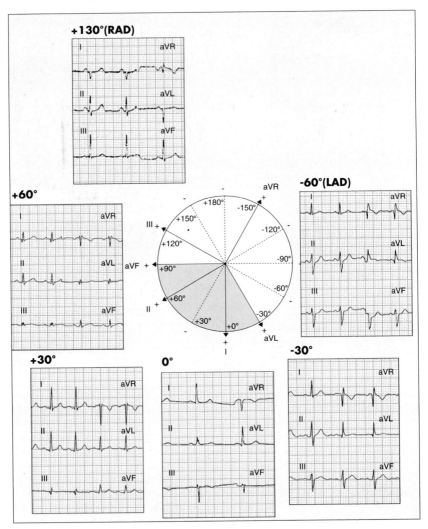

1.4 Mean frontal QRS axis

This is the mean direction of the left ventricular depolarization vector in those leads (I to aVL) which lie in the frontal plane of the heart. It lies at right angles to the lead in which the net QRS deflection is least pronounced. It is quantified using a hexaxial reference system. The QRS axis shows a wide range of normality from −30° to 90°. Thus, despite the different ECG patterns in this illustration only recordings, labelled LAD and RAD, are abnormal because of left and right axis deviation, respectively.

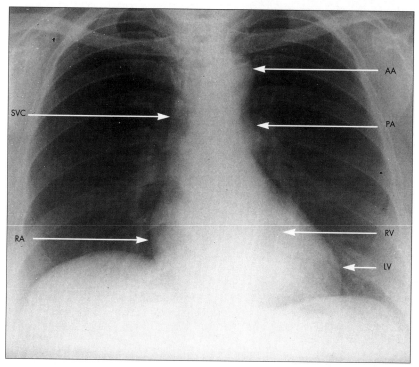

1.5 Chest radiography

This is a postero-anterior projection. Note the heart is not enlarged (cardiothoracic ratio less than 50%) and the lung fields are clear. Cardiac enlargement is caused either by pericardial effusion or by dilatation of the cardiac chambers and great vessels. Heart disease causes lung field abnormalities when left atrial pressure is increased (mitral valve disease, left ventricular failure), resulting in pulmonary congestion. Septal defects may increase pulmonary flow sufficiently to cause pulmonary plethora. Advanced pulmonary vascular disease may reduce pulmonary flow sufficiently to cause oligaemic lung fields with peripheral pruning. SVC = superior vena cava. RA = right atrium. AA = aortic arch. LV = left ventricle. PA = pulmonary artery. RV = right ventricle.

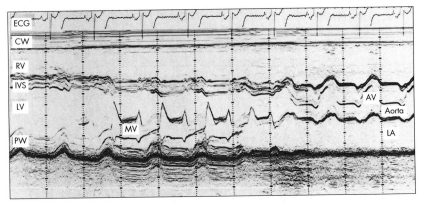

1.6 M-mode echocardiography

This provides a unidimensional 'ice-pick' view through the heart. Continuous recording provides an additional time dimension, permitting appreciation of the dynamic component of the cardiac image. The figure shows a sweep as the transducer is angulated from the left ventricle to the aortic root. The vertical dots are a 1cm scale. CW = chest wall. IVS = interventricular septum. PW = posterior LV wall. MV = mitral valve. AV = aortic valve. LA = left atrium.

1.7a–d Transthoracic two-dimensional echocardiography

This technique provides more detailed structural and dynamic information than the M-mode study. The two-dimensional (2-D) images may be recorded on magnetic tape to provide a 'real time' record of events during the cardiac cycle. The four standard views are shown.

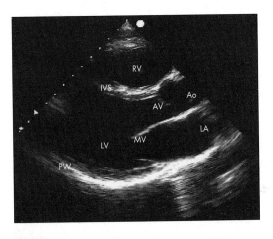

1.7a Parasternal long axis view (diastolic frame).

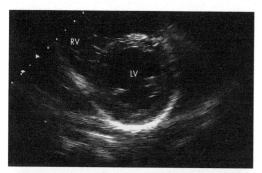

1.7b Parasternal short axis view (papillary muscle level).

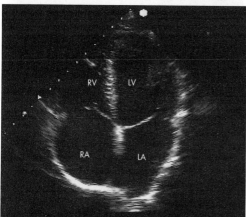

1.7c Apical four-chamber view. TV= tricuspid valve.

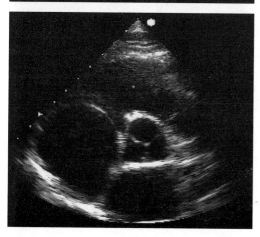

1.7d Parasternal short axis view (aortic valve level). Note that three cusps of the aortic valve are clearly visible in a 'Mercedes Benz'configuration.

1.8a and b Transoesophageal echocardiography

A transducer mounted on a probe is positioned in the oesophagus directly behind the heart. It provides images of exceptional clarity because there are no intervening ribs and the probe is closely applied to the posterior aspect of the heart. Transoesophageal echocardiography (TOE) is particularly useful for imaging the left atrium, aorta and prosthetic heart valves.

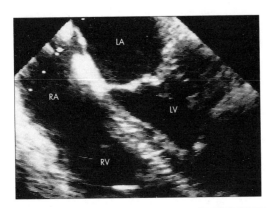

1.8a TOE: four-chamber view commonly used for the diagnosis of atrioseptal defects

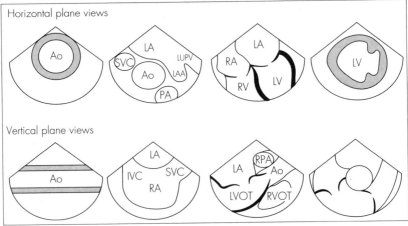

1.8b TOE: these views are routinely obtained during the procedure. Ao= Aorta. SVC=superior vena cava. IVC=interior vena cava. PA=pulmonary artery. RPA=right pulmonary artery. LAA=left atrial appendage. LVOT=left ventricular outflow tract. LUPV=left upper pulmonary vein. RVOT=right venrtricular outflow tract.

1.9a–c Doppler echocardiography

Doppler echocardiography permits evaluation of the direction and velocity of blood flow within the heart and great vessels. It is widely used for measuring the severity of valvular stenosis and for identifying valvular regurgitation and intracardiac shunts caused by septal defects. The introduction of colour flow mapping has been a major technological advance because, by superimposing the colour-coded data on the 2-D echocardiogram, the patterns of flow within the four chambers of the heart can be identified with considerable precision.

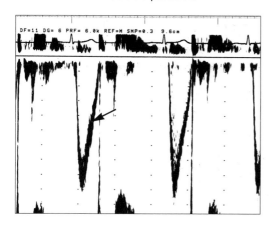

1.9a Normal pulsed-wave Doppler recording from the left ventricular outflow tract. This shows normal laminar flow through the aortic valve (arrowed).

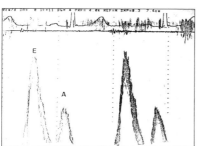

1.9b Normal pulsed-wave Doppler recording of flow across the mitral valve. The early (E wave) and atrial (A wave) components are clearly distinguishable.

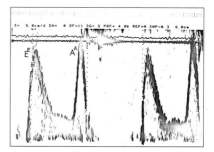

1.9c Many factors affect the ratio between the atrial (A wave) and early (E wave) components of the transmitral Doppler signal. In this example, the Doppler signal in an elderly patient is shown. Note that the A:E ratio is increased and the A wave is larger than the E wave.

1.10a–c Myocardial perfusion imaging

This is used for diagnosis of coronary artery disease. The patient is exercised and, after intravenous injection with a radioisotope, is imaged under a gamma camera. ^{201}Tl is used most commonly but the more recently introduced ^{99m}Tc-labelled MIBI provides better image quality. In the normal heart, isotope is distributed homogeneously throughout the left ventricular myocardium according to coronary perfusion but in coronary artery disease, perfusion defects occur in the distribution of the diseased arteries. Examples of normal ^{99m}Tc MIBI perfusion images are shown. Distribution of isotope is, in all cases, homogeneous. Both left and right ventricles are clearly visible.

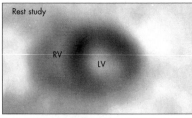

1.10a Normal ^{99m}Tc MIBI perfusion scintiscan: short axis view. Note that isotope is distributed homogeneously throughout the left ventricular myocardium at rest and during exercise, reflecting normal myocardial perfusion.

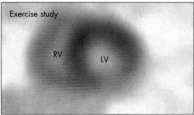

1.10b Normal ^{99m}Tc MIBI perfusion scintiscan: vertical long axis view. Again, isotope is distributed homogeneously throughout the left ventricular myocardium at rest and during exercise, reflecting normal myocardial perfusion.

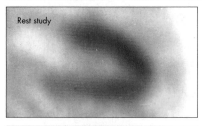

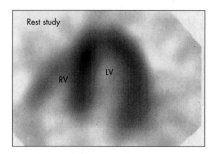

Rest study

RV LV

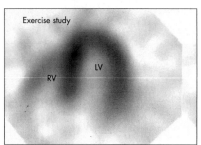

Exercise study

LV
RV

1.10c Normal ^{99m}Tc MIBI perfusion scintiscan: horizontal long axis view. Again, isotope is distributed homogeneously throughout the left ventricular myocardium at rest and during exercise, reflecting normal myocardial perfusion.

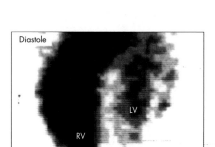

Diastole

LV
RV

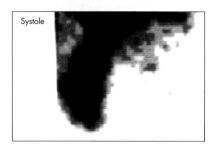

Systole

1.11 Radionuclide ventriculography

This is used for assessment of ventricular function. Red cells labelled with ^{99m}Tc are injected and allowed to equilibrate within the blood pool. The ventricular chambers are imaged with a gamma camera which records peaks and troughs of radioactivity during diastole and systole, respectively. This permits construction of a dynamic ventriculogram which may be used to examine ventricular wall motion and chamber dimensions. In this example, the right and left ventricles are clearly visible. The ventricular cavity is small and during systole contracts vigorously.

1.12a–d Pulmonary scintigraphy

Simultaneous ventilation and perfusion scintigrams (anterior and posterior projections) are shown. Inhaled ^{133}Xe and injected ^{99m}Tc should normally be distributed homogeneously throughout both lung fields, as shown here. Pulmonary embolism produces perfusion defects but does not affect the ventilation scan. Thus, the finding of scintigraphic perfusion defects not matched by ventilation defects is highly specific for this disorder (see 13.1 c).

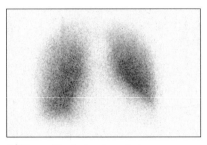

1.12a Ventilation (anterior).

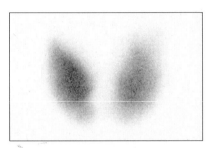

1.12b Perfusion (anterior).

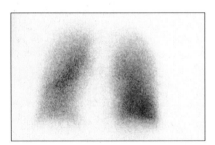

1.12c Ventilation (posterior)

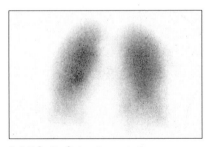

1.12d Perfusion (posterior)

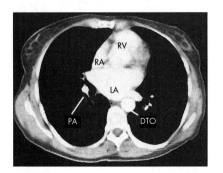

1.13 Computerized tomography

A thoracic tomogram at left atrial level is shown. The vascular spaces have been 'enhanced' by the injection of contrast solution into the bloodstream. DTO = descending thoracic aorta.

1.14a-c Magnetic resonance imaging

Magnetic resonance imaging (MRI) represents a quantum leap forward in terms of image quality (and cost!). It has already found an important role in the diagnosis of aortic dissection. Other potential applications include assessment of myocardial perfusion using paramagnetic contrast agents and identification of histological and metabolic disorders of the myocardium. The realization of this exciting potential will ensure an important role for MRI in clinical cardiology.

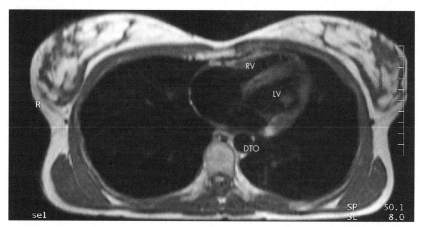

1.14a Normal MRI: transverse section through chest.

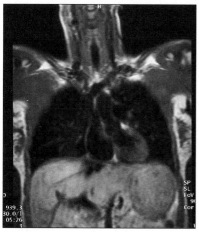

1.14b Normal MRI: coronal section.

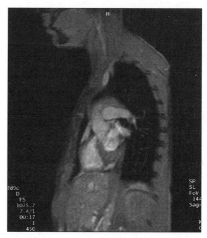

1.14c Normal MRI: sagittal section.

1.15–1.17 Coronary arteriography

This remains the only means of imaging the coronary arteries. The catheter, introduced into the arterial circulation, is directed into the ascending aorta and positioned in the left then right coronary ostia. Contrast material injected through the catheter provides radiographic images of the coronary arteries.

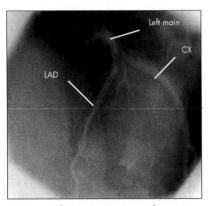

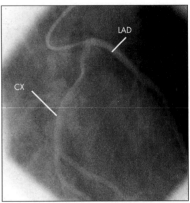

1.15a Left coronary artery: Left anterior oblique (LAO) projection. The left main coronary artery gives two major branches, the left anterior descending (LAD) and circumflex (CX) coronary arteries which supply the anterior and lateral walls of the heart, respectively.

1.15b Left coronary artery: right anterior oblique (RAO) projection.

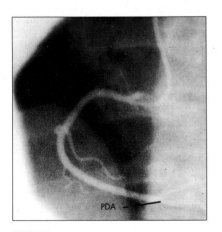

1.15c Right coronary artery: LAO projection. Approximately 85% of the population have a 'right dominant' coronary circulation, in which the right coronary artery gives the posterior descending artery (PDA), supplying the inferior wall of the heart.

1.16a–c In approximately 15% of the population, the posterior descending artery supplying the inferior wall of the heart arises from the circumflex coronary artery. This is termed a 'left dominant circulation'.

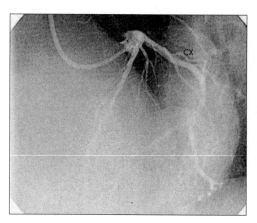

1.16a Left coronary artery. LAO projection. Note the very large circumflex (CX) coronary artery in this left dominant circulation.

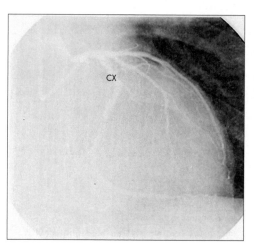

1.16b Left coronary artery. RAO projection. The very large circumflex (CX) coronary artery supplying the posterior descending branch is clearly visible.

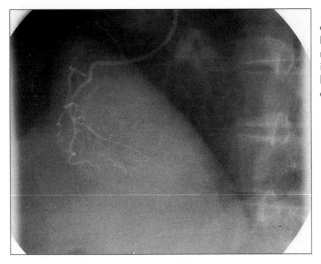

1.16c Right coronary artery: LAO projection. The right coronary artery is diminutive in this left dominant circulation.

1.17a and b Coronary anomalies

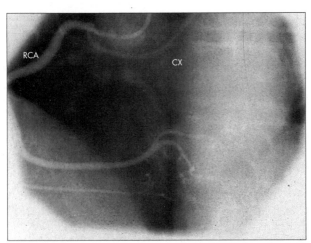

1.17a Anomalous origin of the circumflex artery from the right coronary ostium. This is the most common coronary anomaly, affecting approximately 0.7% of the population.

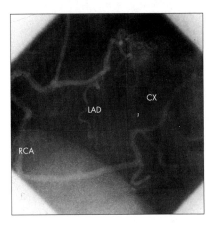

1.17b Much less common is 'single coronary artery', in which the entire coronary supply originates from a single ostium in either the right coronary sinus (as in this example) or the left coronary sinus.

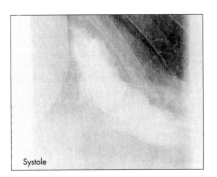

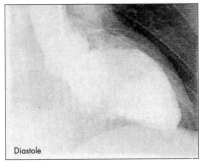

1.18 Left ventriculogram: RAO projection
A catheter has been passed from the ascending aorta through the aortic valve into the left ventricular cavity. These are systolic and diastolic frames from a cine angiogram performed during injection of contrast material. In this normal study, the left ventricle is contracting vigorously with an ejection fraction in excess of 60%.

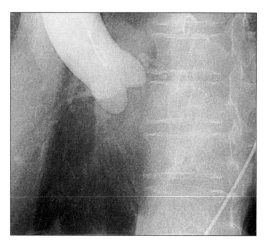

1.19 Aortic root angiogram: LAO projection

The catheter has been pulled back across the aortic valve into the aortic root. Contrast injection shows a normal ascending aorta with coronary arteries clearly visible. Note the aortic valve is competent and there is no regurgitation of contrast backwards into the left ventricle.Compare with figure 5.12.

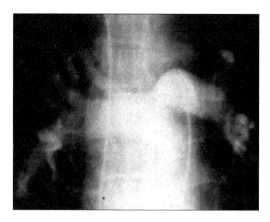

1.20 Pulmonary angiography

A catheter has been guided through the right side of the heart and positioned in the main pulmonary artery. Rapid injection of contrast solution produces opacification of the arterial tree throughout both lung fields. The symmetrical distribution of contrast without filling defects rules out pulmonary embolism.

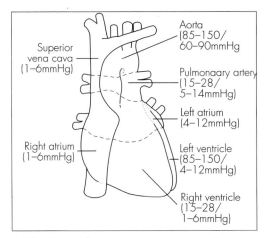

Aorta
(85–150/
60–90mmHg

Superior
vena cava
(1–6mmHg)

Pulmonaary artery
(15–28/
5–14mmHg)

Left atrium
(4–12mmHg)

Right atrium
(1–6mmHg)

Left ventricle
(85–150/
4–12mmHg)

Right ventricle
(15–28/
1–6mmHg)

1.21 Normal pressure measurements within the heart and great vessels

These can be obtained by a fluid-filled balloon-tipped catheter attached to a pressure transducer. Right-sided pressures are obtained with the catheter directed by the venous route into the right atrium and then through the right ventricle into the pulmonary artery. Left-sided pressures are obtained with the catheter directed by the arterial route into the ascending aorta and then backwards through the aortic valve into the left ventricle. Left atrial pressure is usually measured indirectly using the pulmonary artery wedge pressure because access to the left atrium is difficult. This is obtained during right heart catheterization by advancing the catheter distally into the pulmonary arterial tree until the tip wedges in a small branch. The wedge pressure recorded at the catheter tip is a more or less accurate measure of the left atrial pressure transmitted backwards through the pulmonary veins and capillaries.

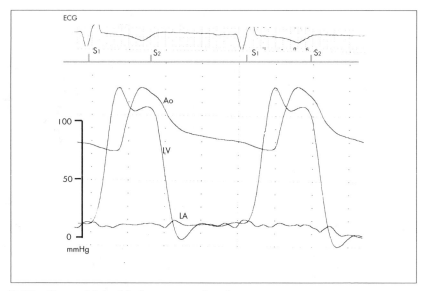

1.22 Normal left-sided pressure signals

Simultaneous recordings of the aortic, left ventricular and left atrial pressure signals are shown. At the end of diastole, after atrial contraction, the sharp rise in left ventricular pressure forces the mitral valve to close which generates the first heart sound(S1). As left ventricular pressure rises above aortic pressure, the aortic valve opens to allow ejection of blood. After this, the pressures in the left ventricle and aorta remain equal and superimposed until the aortic valve closes which generates the first component of the second heart sound (S2). Throughout diastole the decline in aortic pressure is relatively gradual as blood runs off into the peripheral circulation. Left ventricular pressure, on the other hand, falls rapidly and, as it drops below left atrial pressure, the mitral valve opens to allow ventricular filling. This checks the decline in left ventricular pressure which rises slowly until the onset of systole leads to closure of the mitral valve and initiates another cycle.

1.23a and b Right heart catheterization

This can be performed at the bedside using a catheter with a terminal balloon. After introduction of the catheter into a central vein, the balloon is inflated and flow-guided through the right side of the heart into the pulmonary artery.

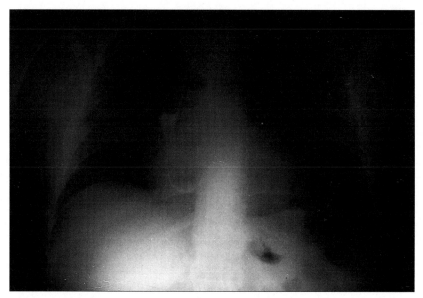

1.23a The catheter is seen lying across the right-sided cardiac chambers with the tip in the pulmonary artery. The terminal balloon (inflated with contrast material to improve visualization) is wedged in a branch artery to record the pulmonary artery wedge pressure which is an indirect measure of left atrial pressure (see 1.21).

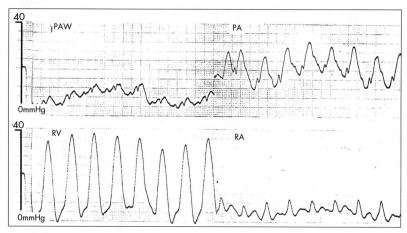

1.23b Pressure signals recorded from a balloon tipped catheter as it is withdrawn from the pulmonary artery into the right atrium. Note how the pressure waveform changes as the catheter is withdrawn through the right side of the heart. Note also the phasic changes in pressure during respiration. PAW = pulmonary artery wedge pressure. RV = right ventricular pressure. RA = right atrial pressure. PA = pulmonary artery pressure.

2.

Signs of Heart Disease

2.1a–h Inspection of the patient

The cardiac examination should start with a general inspection of the patient noting the body habitus, musculoskeletal abnormalities, congenital anomalies and skin lesions.

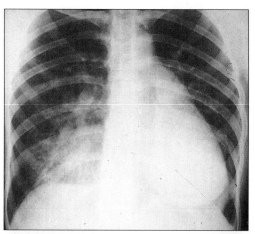

2.1a(i) Chest xray (postero-anterior projection). Pectus excavatum is a common deformity which can displace the heart into the left side of the chest and distort the left ventricular outflow tract resulting in an 'innocent' ejection murmur on auscultation. The displacement of the heart may give a spurious impression of cardiac enlargement as shown in this chest xray.

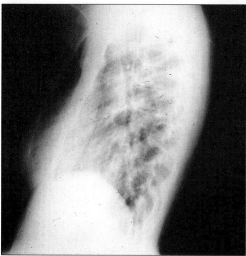

2.1a(ii) Pectus excavatum: chest radiograph (lateral view). The depressed sternum is clearly visible in this projection, compressing the heart against the spinal column.

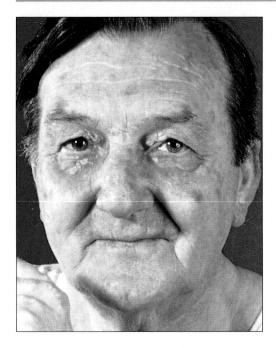

2.1b Cutaneous stigmata of hypercholesterolaemia. Xanthelasmata are clearly visible around the eyes but are not specific for hypercholesterolaemia. Much more specific are tendon xantheiasmata which, in this example, are visible on the knuckles of the hand.

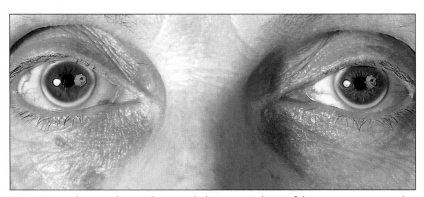

2.1c Corneal arcus. This can be regarded as a normal part of the ageing process and is a nonspecific finding. However, in young patients the presence of a corneal arcus is more predictive of hypercholesterolaemia, particularly when it is eccentric.

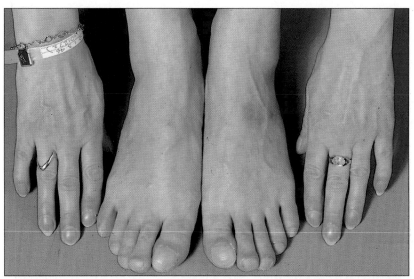

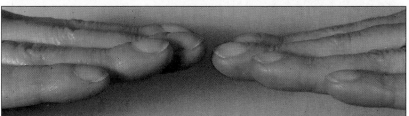

2.1d and e Digital clubbing. Congenital cyanotic heart disease is now the only important cardiac cause of clubbing. Rarely, it may be a manifestation of infective endocarditis.

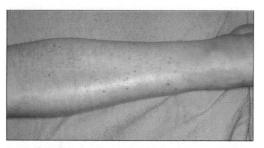

2.1f Diffuse Vasculitic rash. This occurs commonly in infective endocarditis when it is a manifestation of immune complex deposition in the skin.

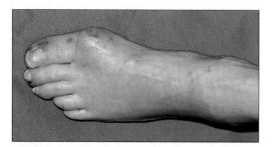

2.1g(i) Discrete Vasculitic rash. Occasionally vasculitic legions are discrete as in this example.

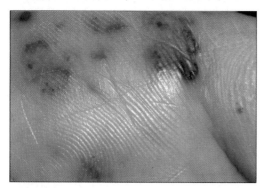

2.1g(ii) Discrete Vasculitic rash. This is a close up of the lesions shown above.

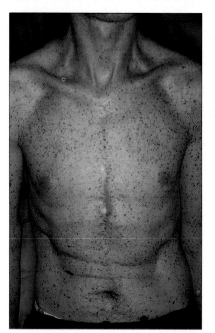 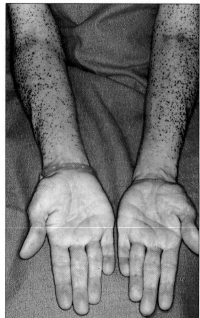

2.1h(i) and (ii) Leopard syndrome. Occasionally patients presenting with cardiovascular disorders have the stigmata of specific congenital disorders. The Leopard syndrome is a rare single-gene defect associated with a complex of congenital malformations. Cutaneous manifestations are the deeply pigmented lentigines shown in these illustrations. Cardiac abnormalities consist of conduction defects and pulmonary stenosis. Other single-gene disorders, including Holt–Oram syndrome and Kartagener's syndrome, are shown in Chapter 11.

2.2a and b Cyanosis

Recognition of cyanosis is particularly important during the cardiac examination.

Cardiac causes of cyanosis			
	Pathophysiology	**Physiological finding**	**Pathological finding**
Peripheral cyanosis (skin and lips)	Desaturation of blood in vasoconstricted cutaneous circulation	Cold exposure	Heart failure
Central cyanosis	Desaturation of arterial blood	Never physiological	Pulmonary oedema
			Cyanotic congenital heart disease

2.2a Cardiac causes of cyanosis are summarized in this table.

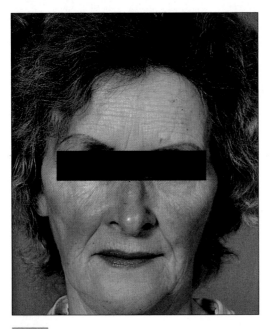

2.2b Mitral facies. The cyanotic discoloration of the cheeks is commonly present in long standing mitral stenosis but is not specific for this condition. The cyanosis is usually attributed to low cardiac output and vasoconstriction.

2.3a–g Causes of an irregular pulse

The radial pulse is examined for rate and rhythm. Normal sinus rhythm is regular. If the pulse is irregular, accurate measurement of heart rate requires auscultation at the cardiac apex (see 2.4). Common causes of irregular pulse are shown.

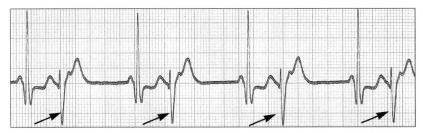

2.3a   Ventricular ectopic beats (arrowed) in bigeminal rhythm.

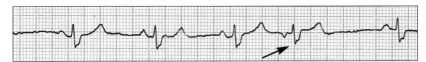

2.3b   Atrial ectopic beat (arrowed) from a low atrial focus.

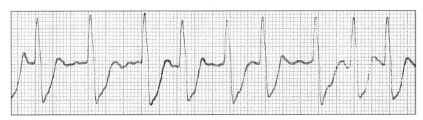

2.3c   Atrial fibrillation.

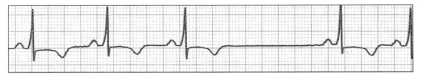

2.3d   Sinus pause. After the second sinus beat there is a long pause.

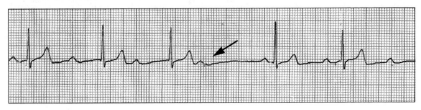

2.3e 2° Atrioventicular block (type 1). The non–conducted P wave is arrowed.

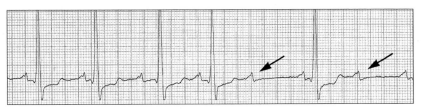

2.3f 2° Atrioventicular block (type 2). The non–conducted P waves are arrowed.

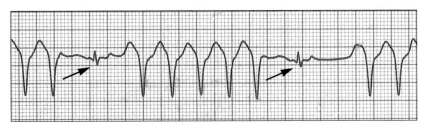

2.3g Paroxysmal ventricular tachycardia. Only 2 sinus beats are seen (arrowed), interrupted by short paroxysms of ventricular tachycardia.

2.4a and b   Pulse rate and blood pressure: effects of an irregular pulse

If diastole is very short, ventricular filling may be critically reduced, such that the pulse pressure generated by systolic contraction is inadequate for palpation at the wrist. For this reason, accurate rate assessment requires auscultation at the cardiac apex when the pulse is irregular.

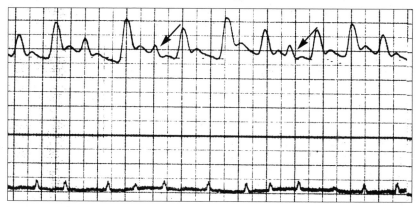

2.4a   Atrial fibrillation. Simultaneous recordings of the ECG and radial artery pressure are shown. Beats following very short diastolic intervals (arrowed) do not generate sufficient pressure for palpation at the wrist.

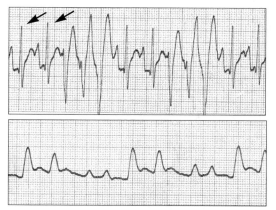

2.4b   Paroxysmal ventricular tachycardia. Simultaneous recordings of the ECG and radial artery pressure signal. Note that the blood pressure generated by sinus beats (arrowed) is normal but during ventricular tachycardia it drops. Again, this is because during the arrhythmia, ventricular filling is inadequate partly because of the rapid rate and partly because of the loss of synchronized atrial activity.

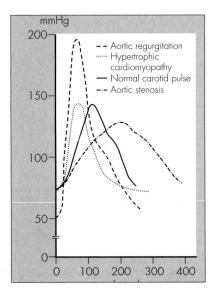

2.5 Pulse character

Although heart rate can usually be assessed by palpation of the radial pulse, pulse character is best assessed by palpation of the carotid artery, the pulse closest to the heart. Waveform is determined principally by the rate of the carotid upstroke. Note in aortic regurgitation, the upstroke is rapid and followed by abrupt diastolic 'collapse'. In hypertrophic cardiomyopathy, the upstroke is also rapid and the pulse has a 'jerky' character. In aortic stenosis the upstroke is slow with a 'plateau'.

2.6a and b   Other abnormalities of the arterial pulse

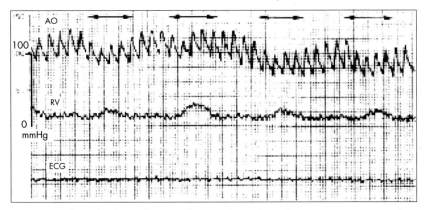

2.6a   Paradoxical pulse and Kussmaul's sign. These physical signs occur in tamponade and pericardial constriction. In this example, pericardial effusion (evidenced by the small voltage deflections on the ECG) has caused tamponade. Respiratory fluctuations in the aortic (AO) and right atrial (RA) pressure signals are seen. During inspiration (arrowed), right atrial pressure rises (Kussmaul's sign) because the increase in venous return cannot be accommodated in the constricted right ventricle. Simultaneously, aortic pressure falls (pulsus paradoxus) because the normal inspiratory increase in right ventricle output is prevented.

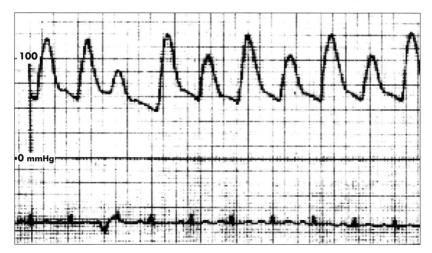

2.6b Alternating pulse. This always indicates advanced left ventricular disease. The alternating high and low systolic peaks are particularly prominent in the beats that follow an extrasystole (as in this example) and can often be detected by palpating the carotid pulse. The mechanism of pulsus alternans is unknown.

2.7 Jugular venous pulse: waveform

The jugular venous pulse (JVP) should be assessed with the patient reclining at 45°. It has a flickering character caused by the 'a' and 'v' waves (see page 34).

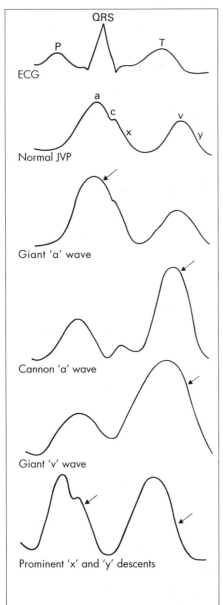

ECG   Electrical events precede mechanical events in the cardiac cycle. Thus, the P wave (atrial depolarizaton) and QRS complex (ventricular depolarization) precede the 'a' and 'v' waves, respectively, of the JVP.

Normal JVP (see 1.23b). The 'a' wave, produced by atrial systole, is followed by the 'x' descent interrupted by the small 'c' wave marking tricuspid valve closure. Atrial pressure then rises again ('v' wave) as the atrium fills passively during ventricular systole.

Giant 'a' wave (arrowed, see 13.3e). Forceful atrial contraction against a stenosed tricuspid valve or a noncompliant hypertrophied right ventricle produces an unusually prominent 'a' wave.

Cannon 'a' wave (arrowed, see 9.6d). This is caused by atrial systole against a closed tricuspid valve. It occurs when atrial and ventricular rhythms are dissociated (complete heart block, ventricular tachycardia) and marks coincident atrial and ventricular systole.

Giant 'v' wave (arrowed, see 5.29a). This is an important sign of tricuspid regurgitation. The regurgitant jet produces pulsatile systolic waves in the JVP.

Prominent 'x' and 'y' descents (arrowed, see 6.11d). These occur in constrictive pericarditis and give the JVP an unusually dynamic appearance. In tamponade, only the 'x' descent is usually exaggerated.

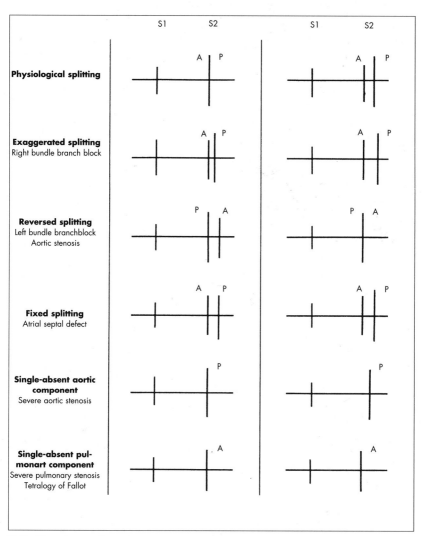

2.8 Heart sounds

The 1st sound, representing mitral and tricuspid closure, is usually single but the aortic and pulmonary components of the 2nd sound normally split during inspiration as increased venous return delays right ventricular emptying. Abnormal splitting of the 2nd heart sound is an important sign of heart disease.

Third and fourth heart sounds (S3 and S4)

	Normal findings	Pathological findings
S3	Age <35 Pregnancy	LVF Mitral regurgitation Ventrical septal defect Aneamia Fever Thyrotoxicosis
S4	Age >70	Hypertension Aortic stenosis Hypertrophic cardiomyopathy Myocardial infarction

2.9 3rd and 4th heart sounds

These low frequency added heart sounds are best heard to the cardiac apex with the bell of the stethoscope. They are associated with rapid ventricular filling which occurs early in diastole (3rd sound [S3]) after mitral and tricuspid valve opening and again late in diastole (4th sound [S4]) as a result of atrial contraction. When present they give a characteristic gallop to the cardiac rhythm. Phonocardiographic recordings of S3 and S4 are shown in 4.7a and 6.6b.

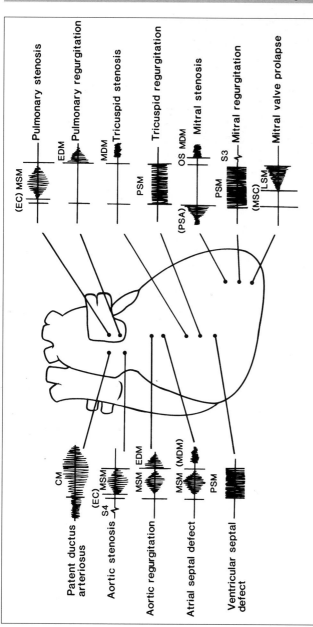

2.10 Heart murmurs

These are caused by turbulent flow within the heart and great vessels and may indicate valve disease or septal defects. Heart murmurs (defined by loudness, quality, location, radiation and timing) may be depicted graphically as shown in this illustration. CM = continuous murmur. EC = ejection click. EDM = early diastolic murmur. LSM = late systolic murmur. MDM = mid-diastolic murmur. MSC = mid-systolic click. MSM = mid-systolic murmur. OS = opening snap. PSA = presystolic accentuation of murmur. PSM = pan-systolic murmur. Parentheses indicate those auscultatory findings that are not constant.

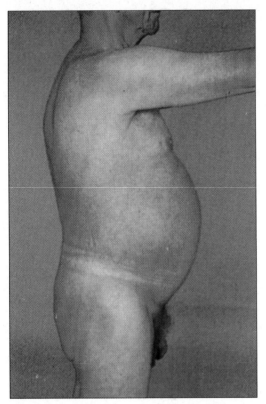

2.11 Salt and water retention: ascites

Salt and water retention is one of the cardinal manifestations of heart failure. As plasma volume expands, central venous pressure and capillary hydrostatic pressure rise, causing oedema fluid to accumulate in the interstitial space. The effect of gravity on capillary hydrostatic pressure ensures that oedema is most prominent around the ankles in the ambulant patient and over the sacrum in the bedridden patient. In advanced heart failure, oedema may involve the legs, genitalia and trunk. Transudation into the peritoneal cavity produces ascites as seen in this illustration. Pleural and pericardial effusions may also develop.

3.

Coronary Artery Disease

3.1a and b Contrast echocardiography to show regional distribution of coronary supply

Territories supplied by the three major coronary arteries are highly circumscribed, the left anterior descending artery supplying the anterior wall, the circumflex artery the lateral wall, and the right coronary artery the inferior wall of the left ventricle. The regional distribution of coronary flow has important implications for electrocardiography and diagnostic imaging because, generally speaking, patients with coronary heart disease show *regional* electrocardiographic or wall motion abnormalities. In these contrast echocardiograms, agitated saline solution was injected first into the left coronary artery (LCA) and then into the right coronary artery (RCA).

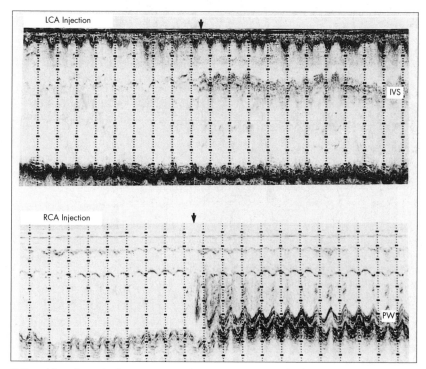

3.1a M-mode study (low gain control). Injections (arrowed) of agitated saline into the left and right coronary arteries cause the interventricular septum (IVS) and posterior wall, (PW) respectively, to 'light up' according to the regional distribution of flow.

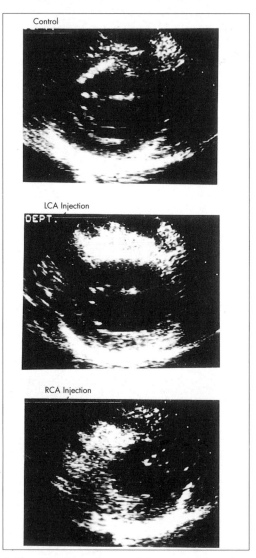

Control

LCA Injection

RCA Injection

3.1b 2-D echocardiogram (left parasternal view). Again, the gain control is low but the left coronary injection 'lights up' the anterior wall of the left ventricle whereas the right coronary injection 'lights up' the posterior wall and the inferior septum.

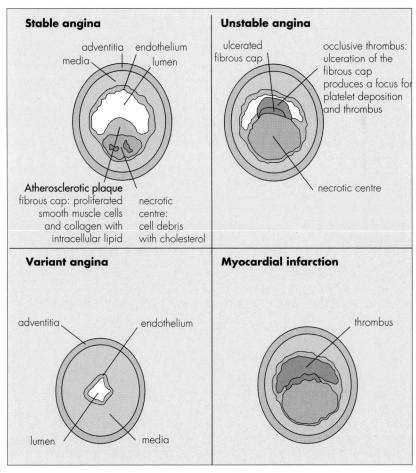

Stable angina

adventitia endothelium
media lumen

Atherosclerotic plaque
fibrous cap: proliferated   necrotic
smooth muscle cells   centre:
and collagen with   cell debris
intracellular lipid   with cholesterol

Unstable angina

ulcerated   occlusive thrombus:
fibrous cap   ulceration of the
fibrous cap
produces a focus for
platelet deposition
and thrombus

necrotic centre

Variant angina

adventitia   endothelium

lumen   media

Myocardial infarction

thrombus

3.2 Coronary syndromes: clinicopathological correlates

The atherosclerotic plaque is the pathological hallmark of coronary artery disease and is responsible directly or indirectly for its ischaemic and thrombotic manifestations. In stable angina, the smooth endothelialized plaque may obstruct coronary flow sufficiently to produce myocardial ischaemia, experienced by the patient as angina. The abrupt rupture of an atheromatous plaque provides a focus of platelet deposition and thrombosis. In unstable angina, the thrombus is subocclusive and causes intense myocardial ischaemia. In myocardial infarction, the thrombus is occlusive, completely obstructing coronary flow. Variant angina is an unusual syndrome of coronary spasm usually associated with atheromatous coronary artery disease. In up to 30% of patients, however, the artery is normal.

3.3a–d   Exercise ECG leads V4–V6

The exercise ECG provides two different types of information in patients with suspected coronary artery disease.

Diagnostic information: exertional tachycardia-increased myocardial oxygen demand. In patients with coronary artery disease, the demand may outstrip coronary supply resulting in regional ischaemia. This causes planar or down-sloping ST segment depression with reversal during recovery.

Prognostic information: a high risk of myocardial infarction or sudden death is indicated by ST depression very early during exercise, an exertional fall in blood pressure or exercise-induced ventricular arrhythmias. Urgent coronary arteriography is required in these patients.

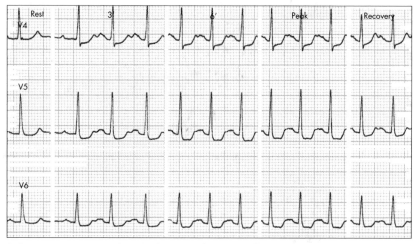

3.3a   Exercise ECG: ischaemic changes. After 3 min of exercise, planar ST depression has developed and at 6min it is more pronounced. The changes reverse during recovery. These changes point to a high probability of coronary artery disease and because they develop early during exercise are prognostically unfavourable.

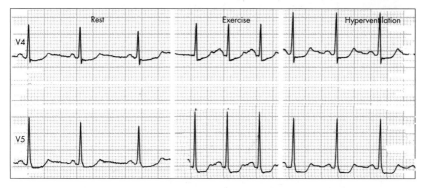

3.3b Exercise ECG: false positive result. The diagnostic accuracy of stress testing is not 100%. False positive and false negative results may occur. In this example, exercise produced ST depression in leads V4–V6. However, angiography showed normal coronary arteries and hyperventilation at a later date produced exactly similar ST segment changes in the absence of significant tachycardia. False positive results like this are particularly common in young women.

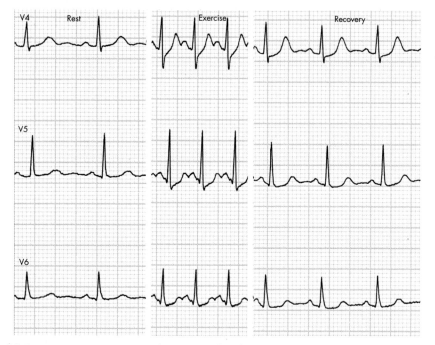

3.3c Exercise ECG: J point depression. The planar ST depression provoked by exercise in patients with coronary artery disease must not be confused with physiological J point depression illustrated in this example. Exercise has caused depression of the junction (J point) between the QRS complex and the ST segment but the ST segment is up-sloping unlike the planar or down-sloping changes seen in patients with coronary artery disease.

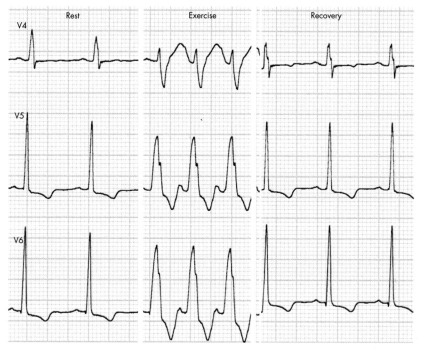

3.3d Exercise ECG: exertional bundle branch block. Occasionally, exercise provokes bundle branch block which makes ST segment analysis difficult or impossible. However, the development of exertional bundle branch block commonly indicates severe underlying coronary artery disease and is usually regarded as an indication for further investigation.

3.4a–d Radionuclide myocardial perfusion imaging

[99m]Technetium–labelled MIBI and [201]thallium are both widely used for myocardial perfusion imaging in the diagnosis of coronary artery disease. They are distributed homogeneously throughout the LV myocardium according to coronary flow and may be imaged under a gamma camera to provide myocardial scintiscans at rest and during exercise-induced ischaemia.

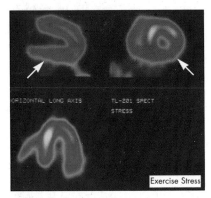
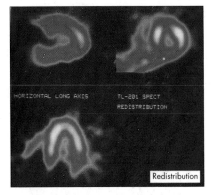

3.4a [201]Thallium scan: partially reversible defect. The scan during exercise-induced ischaemia shows a perfusion defect in the inferior wall (arrowed), strongly suggestive of disease in the right coronary or circumflex arteries. After 3 hour rest, however, the defect has partially disappeared because of the redistribution of isotope. This indicates at least some reversible ischaemia in the territory of the infarct.

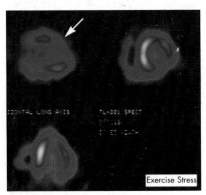
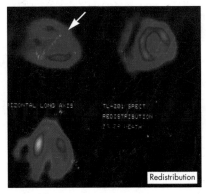

3.4b [201]Thallium scan: fixed defect. A large antero-apical defect (arrowed) is visible not only during exercise but also at rest. Fixed defects of this type indicate infarction in that area. This patient had suffered a left anterior descending coronary occlusion several months before.

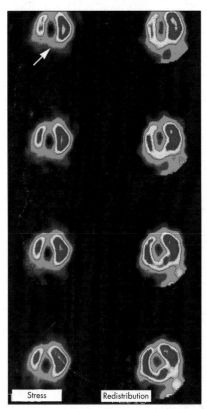 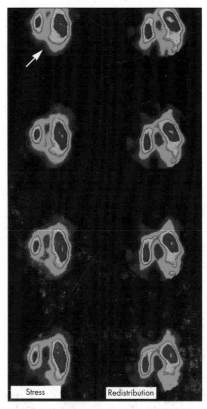

3.4c ²⁰¹Thallium scan: reversible defect. In this short axis view, an inferior wall defect (arrowed) is seen during stress but it largely disappears during rest as the isotope 'redistributes' into the ischaemic area. A smaller fixed defect is seen in the anterior wall indicating infarction in that territory.

3.4d ²⁰¹Thallium scan: reversible defect. In this long axis view (same patient as in **3.4c**), an apical defect (arrowed) is seen during exercise without significant redistribution during rest. This fixed defect indicates that the anterior wall infarct shown in **3.4c** extends down to involve the cardiac apex.

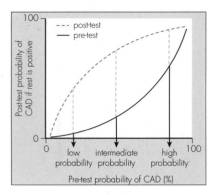

3.5 Probability analysis for coronary artery disease

The reliability of stress testing (ECG or radionuclide perfusion imaging) in the diagnosis of coronary artery disease is not 100% (see 3.3b). Bayes' theory of diagnostic probability states that the predictive accuracy of a positive test will vary according to the probability of coronary disease in the population under study. This is illustrated in the graph shown in this figure. If the pretest probability of coronary disease is very low (e.g. young patients with atypical symptoms) or very high (e.g. more elderly patients with typical symptoms), stress testing is generally unhelpful for diagnostic purposes because a positive test does not increase the probability of disease very much. For this reason, stress testing is best reserved for patients with an intermediate probability of coronary disease based on history, age and sex. In this group, a positive test produces a much larger increase in the probability of coronary disease.

3.6a–i Coronary arteriography

Coronary arteriography remains the generally accepted gold standard for diagnosis of coronary artery disease.

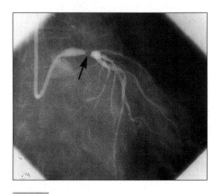

3.6a Left main stem disease (arrowed). This is a very high-risk lesion because the entire left coronary supply is jeopardized and in the event of occlusion, death is almost inevitable.

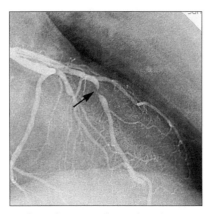

3.6b Left anterior descending disease (arrowed). This tight stenosis threatens the coronary supply to the anterior wall of the left ventricle.

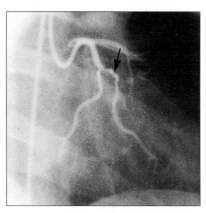

3.6c Circumflex coronary artery disease (arrowed). The disease also involves the origin of the obtuse marginal branch and threatens the coronary supply to the lateral wall of the heart.

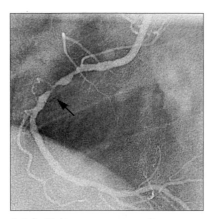

3.6d Right coronary artery disease (arrowed). Serial stenoses in this dominant right coronary artery threaten the supply to the inferior wall of the heart.

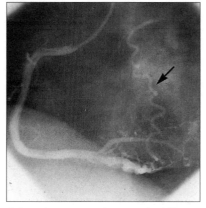

3.6e Coronary occlusion with well-developed collaterals. The left anterior descending coronary artery is occluded. After injection of the right coronary artery, however, collateral flow fills the occluded vessel backwards (arrowed).

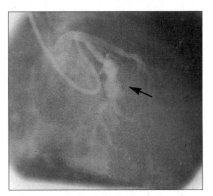

3.6f Ectatic coronary disease. Coronary disease commonly produces arterial ectasia as well as stenosis. Here, there is severe ectasia (arrowed) in a diseased circumflex coronary artery.

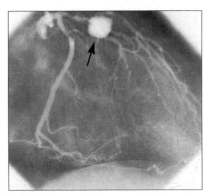

3.6g Aneurysmal coronary disease. This is less common but may occur after angioplasty. Here, there is a large aneurysm (arrowed) involving the proximal part of the left anterior descending coronary artery.

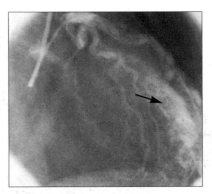

3.6h Congenital AV malformations. These are not uncommon in the coronary circulation and are rarely of clinical importance. However, when large, shunting may be sufficient to cause ischaemia. Here, there is a large AV malformation producing a 'blush' of contrast (arrowed) in close relation to the left anterior descending coronary artery.

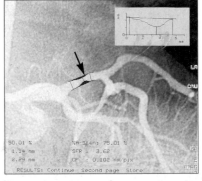

3.6i Quantitative coronary arteriography. The current generation of coronary arteriographic imaging equipment provides computerized assessment of stenosis severity. Here, a tight stenosis in the proximal left anterior descending coronary artery is defined by a process of edge detection and diameter measurement. The severity of the stenosis in relation to the adjacent coronary segment is 75%.

3.7a–d Complications of coronary arteriography

Coronary arteriography is a safe procedure with a mortality risk of less than 1 out of 1000.

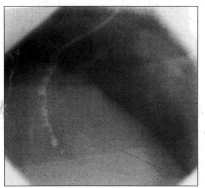

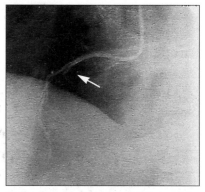

3.7a Intracoronary injection of air. A series of bubbles is clearly visible in the contrast column filling the right coronary artery. If the volume of air is large, it may cause intense ischaemia or cardiac arrest.

3.7b Coronary dissection. The tip of the catheter in the coronary ostium may occasionally traumatize the arterial wall and produce a coronary dissection. In this example, a dissection extending from the catheter tip down the right coronary artery is shown occluding the vessel in its mid-portion (arrowed).

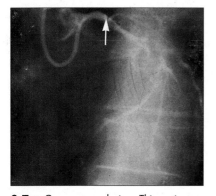

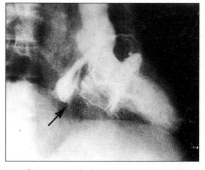

3.7c Coronary occlusion. This patient died during coronary arteriography. The illustration shows a filling defect, almost certainly a thrombus (arrowed), partially occluding the left main coronary artery. The patient had previously suffered a left anterior descending coronary occlusion with anterior myocardial infarction.

3.7d Myocardial penetration. Care must be taken during ventriculography to prevent penetration of the LV myocardium during the contrast injection. Here, the contrast has penetrated the myocardium in a ring around the LV cavity and is seen draining into the coronary sinus (arrowed).

3.8a–i Coronary angioplasty

Percutaneous Transluminal Coronary Angioplasty (PTCA) is increasingly being used to restore coronary patency in symptomatic patients with coronary artery disease. The technique is less invasive and less costly than bypass surgery. Results are best in patients with a proximal stenosis involving only one or two major vessels. The major disadvantage of PTCA is re-stenosis of the artery which occurs in about 30% of patients, nearly always during the first 6 months after the procedure.

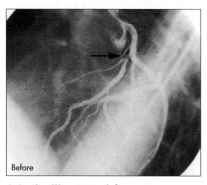

Before

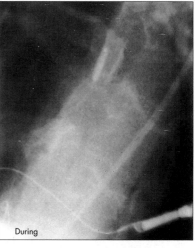

During

3.8a(i)–(iii) PTCA: left anterior descending coronary artery Before PTCA there is a tight stenosis (arrowed) in the left anterior descending coronary artery; the left coronary system is otherwise normal.

(ii) During PTCA, a guide wire has been passed down the diseased vessel and the balloon catheter positioned across the lesion. The balloon is shown inflated in order to dilate the stenosis.

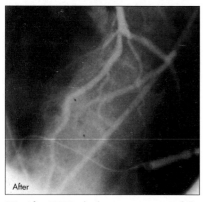

After

(iii) After PTCA, the lesion was successfully dilated and the left anterior descending coronary is now widely patent.

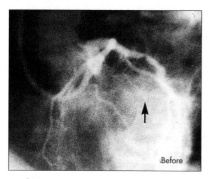

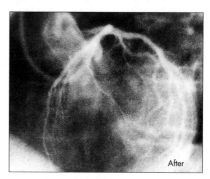

3.8b(i) PTCA: circumflex coronary artery. A discrete eccentric stenosis is shown (arrowed).

3.8b(ii) After the procedure the circumflex coronary artery is widely patent.

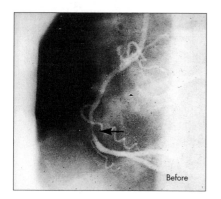

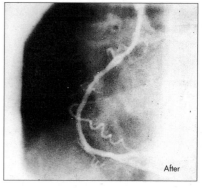

3.8c(i) PTCA: right coronary artery. There is diffuse proximal disease with a tight stenosis (arrowed) in the middle third of the artery.

3.8c(ii) After the procedure, the right coronary artery is widely patent.

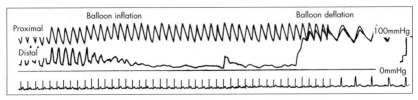

3.8d PTCA: coronary haemodynamic effects. The proximal (aortic) and distal (coronary) pressure signals are shown before, during and after PTCA. Note that before balloon inflation, a significant pressure gradient exists across the stenosis shown by the separation of the proximal and distal signals. Balloon inflation occludes the coronary artery and causes the distal pressure to drop. After balloon deflation with the coronary artery widely patent, distal coronary pressure is restored with abolition of the pressure gradient.

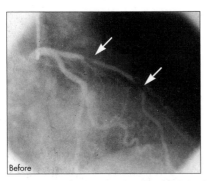
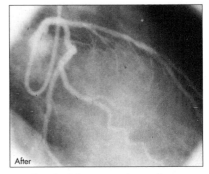

3.8e Complex PTCA. Sequential lesions (arrowed) in the left anterior descending coronary artery before and after successful PTCA.

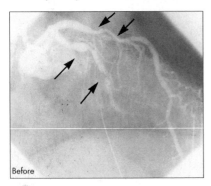
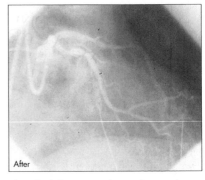

3.8f Complex PTCA. Serial stenoses (arrowed) in the left anterior descending and circumflex coronary arteries are illustrated before and after successful PTCA.

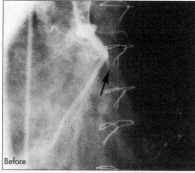

Before

3.8g(i–iii) PTCA: coronary occlusion.
PTCA is successful in only approximately
50% of patients with a completely
occluded coronary artery.
(i) Here, a large obtuse marginal branch
of the circumflex coronary artery was
occluded (arrowed).In a patient who had
previously undergone coronary bypass
surgery (note the sternal sutures).

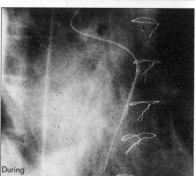

During

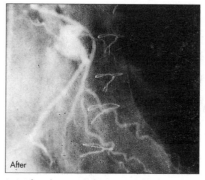

After

(ii) During PTCA, the guide wire and
balloon were successfully directly across the
occlusion

(iii) After the procedure, complete patency
of the branch was restored.

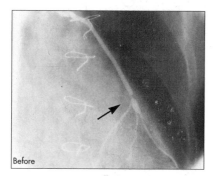

Before

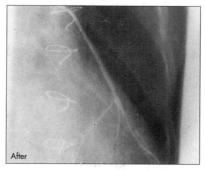

After

3.8h PTCA: vein graft disease. The vein graft to the lateral circumflex artery has a
tight stenosis (arrowed) close to its insertion into the native vessel. After PTCA, the
stenosis is widely dilated and runoff into the native vessel is excellent.

3.8i(i and ii) PTCA: two balloons. Disease involving the bifurcation between a major vessel and its large side branch poses special problems during PTCA. The risk of side branch occlusion an be reduced by simultaneous inflations of balloons in the main vessel and its branch.

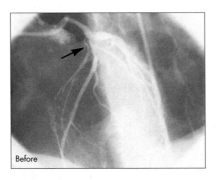

Before

During

3.8i(i) Here, there is severe disease involving the proximal left anterior descending artery and the origin of its first diagonal branch (arrowed).

3.8i(ii) During angioplasty, the balloons were inflated simultaneously in order to preserve patency in both vessels.

3.9a–f   Complications of PTCA

PTCA is successful in over 90% of patients. However, if coronary occlusion occurs during the procedure, there may be the need for urgent coronary bypass surgery if patency cannot be restored using 'bail-out' techniques. Approximately 4% of patients sustain myocardial infarction during angioplasty and about 1% of patients die.

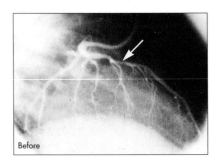

Before

3.9a   Left anterior descending coronary occlusion
(i) Before PTCA, there is a long area of disease in the proximal part of the coronary artery (arrowed).

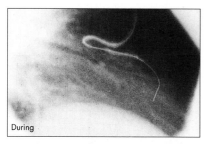

During

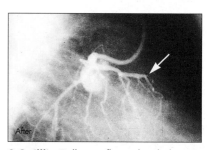

After

3.9a(ii) During the procedure, the guide wire was passed across the diseased segment but has inadvertently entered a septal branch.

3.9a(iii) Balloon inflation has led to complete occlusion of the vessel (arrowed).

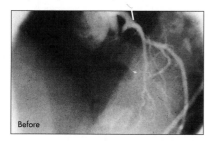

Before

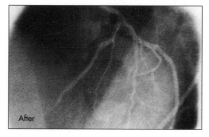

After

3.9b(i) and (ii) Coronary dissection. Dissections of this type often heal spontaneously without further intervention. Increasingly, however, intraluminal stents are being applied in these situations to prevent coronary occlusion (see **3.10a–g**).Before PTCA the left anterior descending coronary artery was occluded (arrowed), after PTCA the vessel was a residual coronary dissection (arrowed)

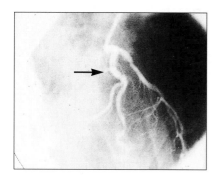

3.9c Coronary dissection. This patient had undergone PTCA of a proximal stenosis in the circumflex coronary artery. The artery (arrowed) is widely patent but a dissection is clearly visible running almost the whole length of the vessel. This is a very unstable situation and in most cases extensive stenting or coronary bypass surgery is necessary to maintain patency of the vessel.

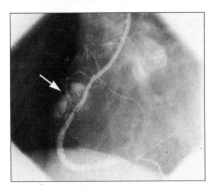

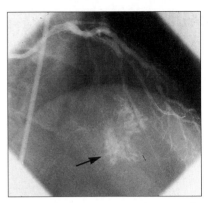

3.9d Coronary rupture. Right coronary PTCA had led to extensive dissection. Stents had already been applied distally but during dilatation of the proximal part of the vessel, rupture occurred with dye extravasating into the pericardial space (arrowed). This situation demands emergency pericardiocentesis and bypass surgery is often necessary.

3.9e Coronary rupture. In this unusual case, PTCA led to rupture of the left anterior descending coronary artery not into the pericardial space but into the right ventricle. Note the 'blush' (arrowed) as contrast material extravasates into the ventricular cavity.

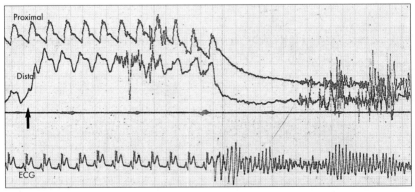

3.9f Ventricular fibrillation (VF). Simultaneous recordings of the proximal and distal coronary arterial pressures are shown during PTCA. After deflation of the balloon (arrowed) the distal coronary pressure rises but the patient goes abruptly into VF with collapse of both pressure signals. Note that the balloon occlusion of the coronary artery produced marked ST elevation on the ECG before the development of VF.

3.10a–f Coronary stenting

Abrupt coronary closure during PTCA and re-stenosis in the first 6 months afterwards remain the major problems with this technique. Aspirin reduces the risk of abrupt thrombotic closure but, to date, no pharmacological interventions have been shown to affect the risk of re-stenosis. The recent introduction of coronary stents, however, has provided an effective 'bail-out' technique for dealing with abrupt coronary closure caused by local dissection; preliminary evidence suggests that stenting may also reduce the incidence of re-stenosis.

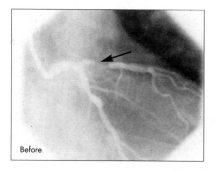
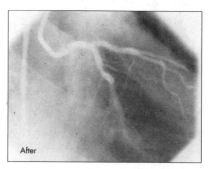

3.10 a Single coronary stent. A tight stenosis (arrowed) in the proximal left anterior descending coronary artery is shown before and after coronary stenting.

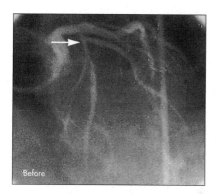
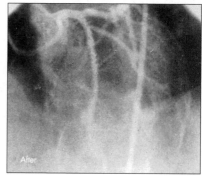

3.10b Sequential stents. A long complex stenosis (arrowed) is shown at the origin of the left anterior descending coronary artery. PTCA produced an unsatisfactory result with local dissection and threatened re-occlusion. After insertion of two sequential intracoronary stents an excellent result was obtained.

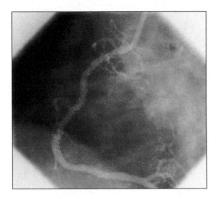

3.10c Multiple stents. PTCA of the proximal part of the right coronary artery produced a long dissection with threatened occlusion. Deployment of four sequential stents produced a good final result.

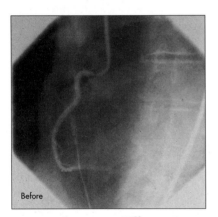

Before

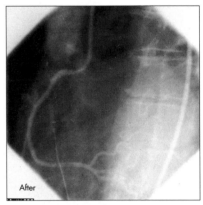

After

3.10d Coronary ostial stent. Coronary ostialial lesions are particularly prone to re-stenosis after conventional PTCA. Before PTCA there is a tight ostial stenosis of the right coronary artery (arrowed). After PTCA, a stent was deployed to maintain patency.

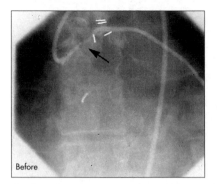

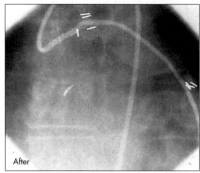

3.10e Coronary vein graft stent. The re-stenosis rate after conventional PTCA is considerably higher for coronary vein grafts compared with native vessels. There is now clear evidence, however, that the use of stents can substantially improve the long term result. Here, there is a long stenosis (arrowed) involving the origin of a graft to the left anterior descending coronary artery. After PTCA the graft was stented to maintain long--term patency.

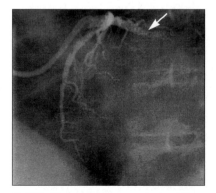

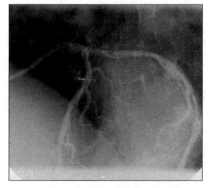

3.10f Thrombotic stent occlusion. Treatment with asprin and other anti–platelet drugs is often recommended after stent deployment to prevent thrombotic occlusion. Here, a stent (arrowed) in the proximal circumflex artery occluded soon after its deployment (left), requiring an emergency return to the catheter laboratory in order to re–open the artery (right).

3.11a–f Intravascular ultrasound

An ultrasound transducer mounted at the tip of a coronary catheter can now be used to provide cross-sectional images of the artery. Intravascular ultrasound (IVUS) is already finding application in coronary angioplasty when 'before and after' images can be used to document satisfactory patency of the vessel.

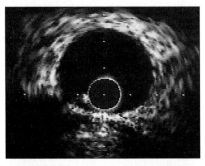

3.11a IVUS: a normal cross-sectional ultrasound scan in a distal segment of the right coronary artery. The ultrasound transducer is clearly visible at the intersection of the horizontal and vertical cm scales.

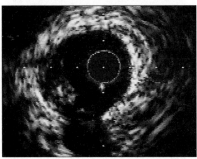

3.11b IVUS: the transducer has been pulled back into a diseased segment of the artery which was recently treated by angioplasty. Atheromatous plaque is visible extending between the 6 o'clock and 9 o'clock positions of the arterial lumen. The plaque has been dissected by the angioplasty procedure, shown by the echo free segment at the 6 o'clock position extending into the arterial wall.

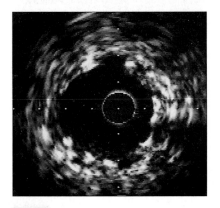

3.11c IVUS: this is the same segment as in **3.11b** after insertion of a coronary stent. The echo-dense struts of the stent are clearly visible around the circumference of the arterial wall.

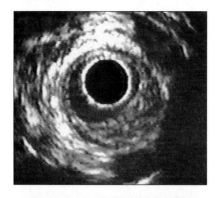

3.11d IVUS: a large semi-lunar coronary plaque extending from the 1 o'clock to the 7 o'clock positions is shown severely reducing the coronary arterial lumen.

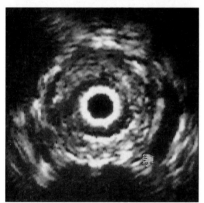

3.11e IVUS: a circumferential plaque after PTCA. Note the clear dissection within the plaque at the 8 o'clock position.

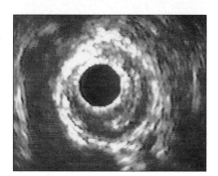

3.11f IVUS: circumferential coronary plaque after PTCA. An extensive area of plaque dissection is seen extending from the 12 o'clock to the 9 o'clock positions. This patient later underwent coronary stenting to maintain patency of the vessel.

3.12a–f Coronary bypass surgery

Coronary artery bypass grafting (CABG) remains the revascularization procedure of choice for many patients, particularly those with extensive three-vessel disease and left main coronary artery disease. In these groups, surgery has been shown to improve not only symptoms but also the long term prognosis.

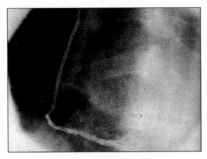

3.12a CABG: vein graft to the posterior descending branch of the right coronary artery.

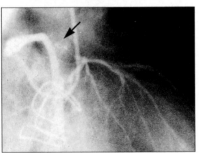

3.12b CABG: a vein graft (arrowed) inserted into the circumflex coronary artery fills the entire coronary system in this patient with left main coronary artery occlusion. The patient had previously undergone valve replacement and the struts of the porcine valve are clearly visible.

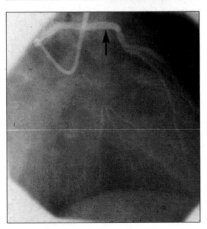

3.12c CABG: a vein graft (arrowed) has been applied 'sequentially' to the left anterior descending coronary artery and its diagonal branch ('jump graft').

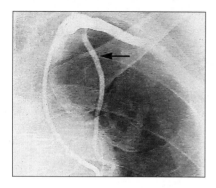

3.12d Left internal mammary artery (LIMA) graft (arrowed).The LIMA has been grafted to the left anterior descending coronary artery. LIMA grafts are now used preferentially for left anterior descending coronary disease because they produce a better long term result than vein grafts which usually occlude within 10 years.

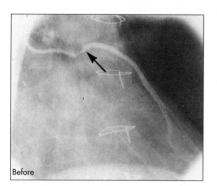

Before

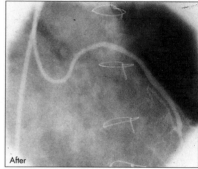

After

3.12e Vein graft disease. Before PTCA there is a tight stenosis (arrowed) at the origin of a left anterior decending coronary vein graft. After PTCA and stent insertion the graft is widely patent.

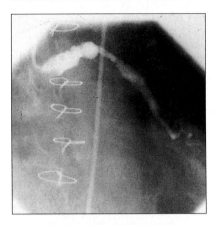

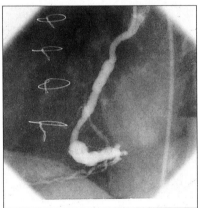

3.12f Vein graft ectasia. As with the native coronary circulation, vein grafts may develop both stenotic and ectatic disease. Here, a left anterior descending coronary vein graft is shown above, and a right coronary vein grafts is shown below. Note the severely ectatic segments proximally in the left anterior descending graft and more distally in the right coronary vein graft.

3.13 Prognosis and coronary artery disease

Coronary artery disease is the most common cause of premature death in the UK. The risk of death is dependent on the extent of the disease and also the severity of left ventricular dysfunction.

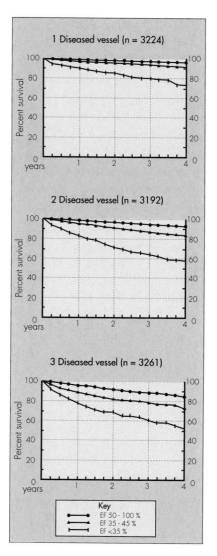

3.13 Survival curves by number of diseased vessels for patients with coronary artery disease treated medically in the registry of the Coronary Artery Surgery Study (CASS). The data are stratified for left ventricular ejection fraction (EF). Note that as the extent of coronary artery disease increases, prognosis deteriorates, patients with 3 vessel disease having the worst prognosis. Similarly, as left ventricular function gets worse, prognosis deteriorates patients with LV ejection fractions<35%, having the worst prognosis.

3.14a and b   Unstable angina: ECG

Patients with unstable angina may present with completely normal ECGs. Typically, however, episodes of unstable chest pain are associated with ST segment or T wave changes.

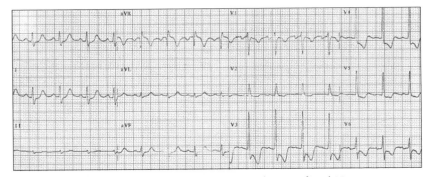

3.14a   The ECG in this patient with unstable angina shows profound ST segment depression extending from V3 to V6 in the area supplied by the left anterior descending coronary artery. ST depression of this type is a bad prognostic sign and is usually regarded as an indication for urgent cardiac catheterization.

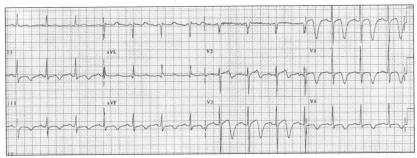

3.14b   In this patient, unstable angina was associated with profound T wave inversion extending from V2 to V6 in the region of the left anterior descending coronary artery.

3.15a–c Unstable angina treated by coronary angioplasty

Revascularization by PTCA or CABG must be considered in all patients with unstable angina, particularly in those who fail to respond rapidly to medical treatment.

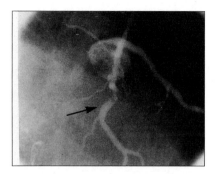

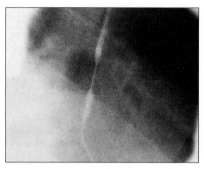

3.15a In this example, the subocclusive coronary thrombus responsible for the unstable presentation is clearly visible (arrowed) as a filling defect in the circumflex coronary artery before PTCA.

3.15b During PTCA the balloon has been inflated across the diseased segment.

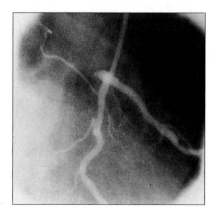

3.15c After PTCA the cicumflex coronary artery is widely patent and the patient exprienced no further chest pain.

3.16a and b Prognosis in unstable angina

There is a significant risk in unstable angina of progression to myocardial infarction and death if the thrombus comes to occlude the coronary artery. Treatment with heparin and aspirin, both of which have a favourable effect on the thrombotic process, have been shown to improve prognosis.

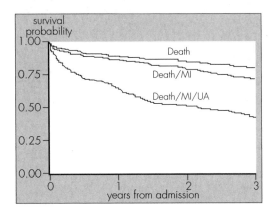

3.16a Survival and event-free survival curves in unstable angina for 544 patients. Event-free survival is shown for major ischaemic end points: myocardial infarction and myocardial infarction or unstable angina.

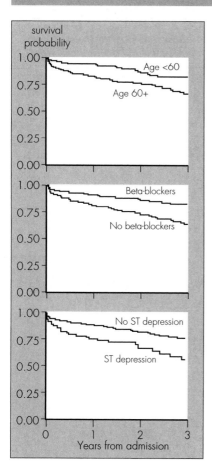

3.16b Infarction-free survival curves for 544 patients with unstable angina are shown. The data show the effects of age, beta blockers and ST depression on prognosis. Note that younger patients usually fare better as do patients treated with beta blockers and those without ST depression on the ECG. (Data from the Newham General Hospital Coronary Care Unit database)

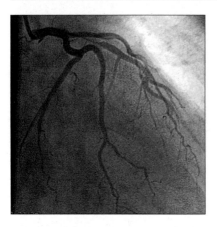

3.17a Variant angina the anatomical substrate. Intense spasm in the proximal left anterior descending coronary artery was shown (arrowed) during diagnostic coronary arteriography in this patient with a long history of intermittent chest pain culminating in anterior mycardial infarction.

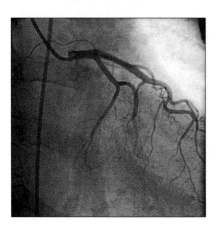

3.17b Variant angina: the response to nitrates. After intracoronary injection of nitrate, the spasm in the proximal left anterior descending coronary artery (see above) resolved, revealing a completely normal coronary circulation.

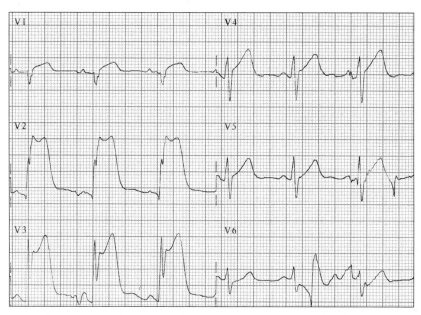

3.18 Variant angina: the electrocardiogram (leads V1–V6). This was ECG-recorded during the coronary arteriograms shown in 3.17. Note the profound ST elevation in leads V1–V4. After intracoronary injection of nitrate, the ECG changes resolved completely.

3.19a and b Diagnosis of acute myocardial infarction

Acute myocardial infarction (AMI) is diagnosed when two of the following three criteria are fulfilled:
• Chest pain
• Regional ST elevation on ECG
• Diagnostic rise in cardiac enzymes

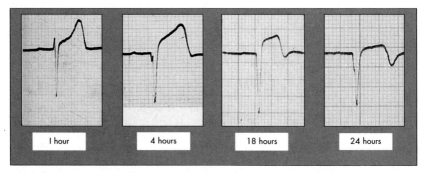

| 1 hour | 4 hours | 18 hours | 24 hours |

3.19a AMI: evolution of ECG changes. Elevation of the ST segment occurs during the first hour of chest pain. The Q wave develops during the subsequent 24 hr and usually persists indefinitely. Within a day of the attack, the ST segment usually returns to the iso-electric line and T wave inversion may occur.

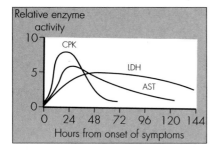

3.19b Time– activity curves for enzyme released from the infarcted myocardium. Serum enzyme activity is expressed in multiples of the upper reference limit.
• Creatine kinase. This is clinically the most useful enzyme. Skeletal muscle is rich in creatine kinase and false positive results are sometimes found in patients who have received intramuscular injections. Greater specificity is provided by the MB iso-enzyme which is specific for the myocardium.
• Aspartate transaminase. Diagnostic value is limited by lack of specificity.
• Lactic dehydrogenase. Diagnostic value is limited by the late peak.

3.20a–d Thrombolytic therapy: effects on diagnostic markers of acute infarction

Thrombolytic therapy has revolutionized the management of AMI. Together with aspirin, it can restore patency of the infarct-related artery. Reperfusion of the threatened myocardium reduces infarct size and improves survival. It is important to recognize the effects that thrombolytic therapy may have on the diagnostic markers of AMI.

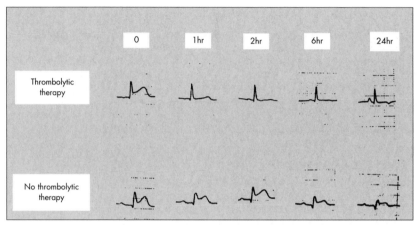

3.20a Thrombolytic therapy and evolution of ECG change: lead 2 in acute inferior myocardial infarction is shown. Thrombolytic therapy produces rapid normalization of ST elevation within an hour of treatment, often without the later development of Q waves. Compare this with the patient who did not receive thrombolytic therapy: there is persistent ST elevation throughout the first 24 hr with loss of R wave and the development of an early Q wave.

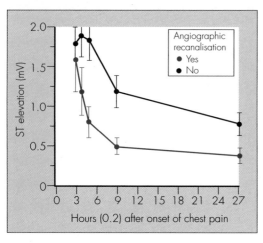

3.20b Thrombolytic therapy: evolution of ST segment change. ST elevation is the ECG hallmark of coronary occlusion. Rapid normalization of ST elevation after thrombolytic therapy reflects successful coronary recanalization. This figure shows the evolution of ST change in two groups of patients, one with successful coronary recanalisation, the other with persistent coronary occlusion shown angiographically. Note how early recanalization produces rapid normalization of ST elevation.

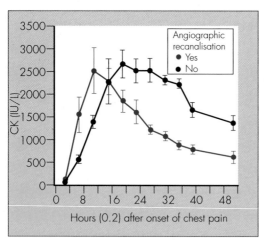

3.20c Thrombolytic therapy: evolution of creatine kinase change. The figure shows the evolution of plasma creatine kinase change early after the onset of chest pain in AMI. The curves are for two groups of patients, one with successful coronary recanalization, the other with persistent coronary occlusion. Note how successful recanalisation produces an early peak in plasma creatine kinase followed by a rapid decline towards normal.

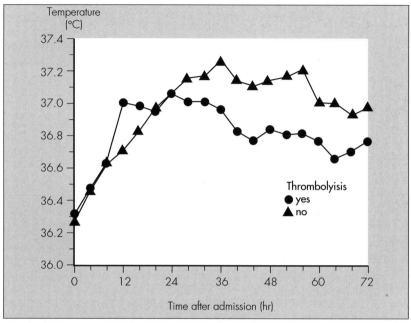

3.20d Thrombolytic therapy: evolution of temperature response. Myocardial infarction produces a low grade pyrexia iin the first 3–4 days caused by the release of pyrogens from the damaged myocardium. The figure shows temperature curves for two groups of patients with AMI; one received thrombolytic therapy, the other did not. Note how thrombolytic therapy is associated with an early peak in temperature (analogous to the early peak in serum creatine kinase shown in 3.20c) and attenuation of the pyrexial response, presumably reflecting reduction in infarct size.

3.21a-e AMI: ECG and infarct location

AMI produces regional changes on the ECG depending on which coronary artery is occluded (see 3.1).

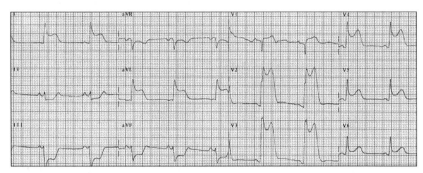

3.21a Acute anterior infarction. ECG 2 hr after the onset of chest pain. ST elevation is evident in leads V1–V6 and also in I and aVL. Note reciprocal ST segment depression in leads II, III and aVF. This pattern usually reflects proximal occlusion of the left anterior descending coronary artery.

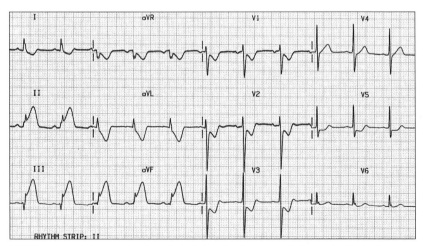

3.21b Acute inferior infarction. ECG 2 hr after the onset of chest pain. Typical changes are evident in leads II, III and aVF. Note reciprocal ST depression in leads I and aVL and also the anteroseptal chest leads (V1–V3). This pattern usually reflects occlusion of the right coronary artery, or alternatively, a dominant circumflex coronary artery.

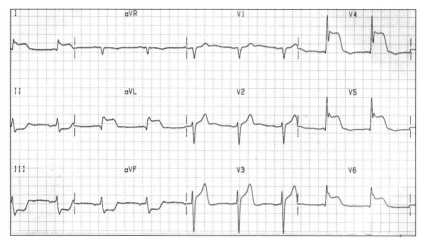

3.21c Acute lateral infarction. ECG 1 hr after the onset of chest pain. Typical changes in the lateral chest leads (V4–V6) and the high lateral limb leads (I and aVL). Note the reciprocal changes in leads II, III and AVF. This pattern usually reflects occlusion of the circumflex coronary artery or, perhaps, a large diagonal branch of the left anterior descending coronary artery.

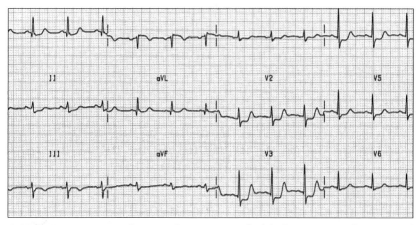

3.21d Acute posterior infarction. The posterior wall of the heart is not well represented on the standard 12 lead ECG. Note the dominant R wave in leads V1 and V2 associated with ST segment depression in the same leads. This pattern usually reflects occlusion of the right coronary artery or, alternatively, a dominant circumflex coronary artery.

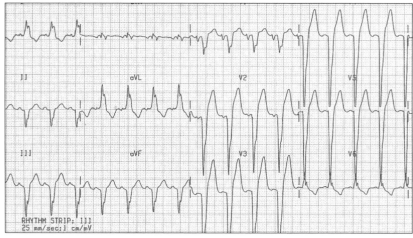

3.21e AMI: left bundle branch block. This ECG pattern may be consistent with AMI but the diagnosis must be made by other means (cardiac enzymes, noninvasive imaging) because the appearances are nonspecific and usual electrocardiographic criteria for AMI cannot be applied. If the diagnosis is confirmed, left bundle branch block always reflects extensive damage to the heart and the prognosis is poor (see 3.26b).

3.22a–c Imaging in AMI

Imaging techniques are rarely helpful for diagnostic purposes in AMI but in difficult cases, where the diagnosis is in doubt, they occasionally provide useful additional information.

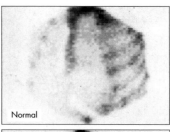
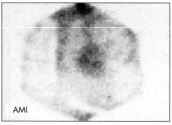

3.22a AMI: hotspot myocardial imaging. ^{99m}Tc pyrophosphate is selectively taken up by acutely infarcted myocardium and may be imaged with a gamma camera. The figure shows scans in a normal patient and a patient with AMI. Note that in the patient with AMI, isotope has become concentrated in a large myocardial infarct revealed as a dense shadow in the left side of the chest. Isotope is also taken up by normal bone and the ribs are clearly visible in both scans.

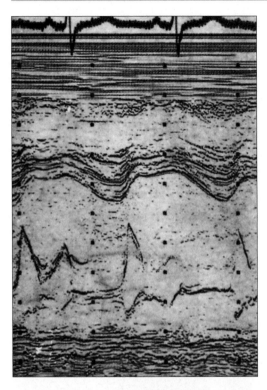

3.22b AMI: M-mode echocardiogram. Akinesis of the posterior wall of the left ventricle with exaggerated motion of the interventricular septum in acute inferior myocardial infarction is shown. Note that regional wall motion abnormalities of this type are not specific for acute infarction but may also occur in patients with old infarction or unstable angina.

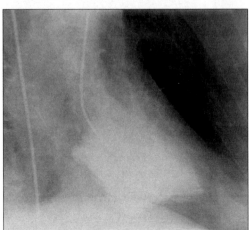

3.22c AMI: left ventriculogram. The angiogram is a mid-systolic frame and shows a localized bulge of the inferior wall in a patient who had recently presented with acute infarction. The coronary arteriogram showed a right coronary occlusion. More patients are now coming to cardiac catheterization in acute myocardial infarction for treatment by direct angioplasty.

3.23a–c Thrombolytic therapy in AMI

Thrombolytic therapy can restore patency of the infarct-related artery in AMI. Reperfusion of the threatened myocardium produces variable salvage within the area at risk, depending largely on the timing of treatment. In general, the earlier thrombolytic therapy is given after the onset of symptoms, the greater the reduction in eventual infarct size.

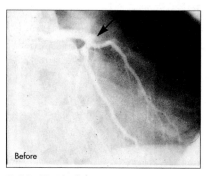

3.23a(i) The left coronary arteriogram taken shortly after presentation with anterior infarction shows a proximal occlusion of the left anterior descending coronary artery (arrowed).

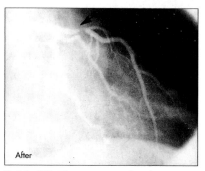

3.23a(ii) Thirty minutes after the administration of streptokinase, luminal patency was restored, although there remains a tight proximal stenosis (arrowed).

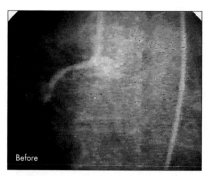

3.23b(i) This right coronary arteriogram, in apatient with acute inferior infarction, shows proximal occlusion, with a filling defect representing thrombus clearly visible in the dye column.

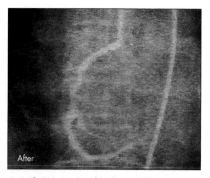

3.23b(ii) Early after thrombolytic therapy, a repeat coronary arteriogram shows recanalisation of the artery but again there is a tight residual stenosis.

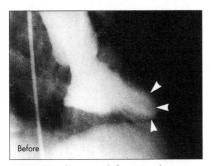

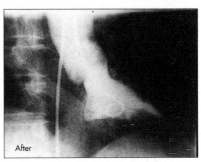

3.23c(i) These are left ventriculograms before and 2 weeks after thrombolytic therapy in acute anterior myocardial infarction caused by left anterior descending coronary arterial occlusion. Note that before thrombolytic therapy there isa large akinetic apical segment (arrowed).

3.23c(ii) However, 2 weeks after thrombolytic therapy contractile function has largely recovered as a result of reperfusion of the ischaemic zone.

3.24 Complications of thrombolytic therapy

Although minor haemorrhagic complications are not uncommon after thrombolytic therapy in AMI, major bleeds are rarer with haemorrhagic stroke occurring in less than 0.1% of patients. Randomized controlled trials have confirmed that the benefits of treatment significantly outweigh the risks. Other complications of thrombolytic therapy include transitory hypotension, minor allergic reactions and occasionally anaphylaxis. These are seen almost exclusively with streptokinase and do not occur with tissue plasminogen activator. Early concerns about 'reperfusion' arrhythmias after thrombolytic therapy have proved largely unfounded. Accelerated idioventricular rhythm is seen commonly but it is of no haemodynamic importance and occurs almost as commonly in patients who do not receive thrombolytic therapy.

3.24 Complications in thrombolytic therapy

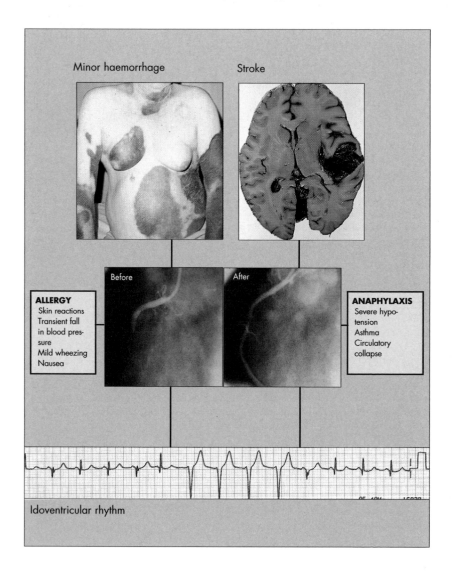

Minor haemorrhage

Stroke

Before

After

ALLERGY
Skin reactions
Transient fall
in blood pres-
sure
Mild wheezing
Nausea

ANAPHYLAXIS
Severe hypo-
tension
Asthma
Circulatory
collapse

Idoventricular rhythm

3.25a–c Primary PTCA in AMI

PTCA may also be used to restore coronary patency in AMI. Clearly, this is only feasible in centres with the appropriate facilities and expertise but the results of comparative trials indicate that the outcome, in terms of recurrent infarction and early mortality, may be better than for thrombolytic therapy. Direct PTCA appears particularly useful for the treatment of cardiogenic shock where mortality can be reduced from 80% to less than 50%.

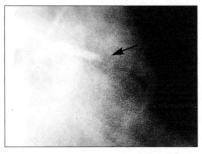

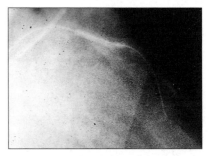

3.25a Proximal occlusion (arrowed) of the left anterior descending coronary artery in a patient presenting with anterior infarction and cardiogenic shock.

3.25b The PTCA balloon has been positioned across the coronary occlusion.

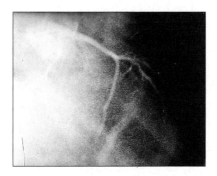

3.25c After PTCA, the coronary artery is widely patent with good runoff into the distal vessel. The patient made a good recovery and survived to be discharged from hospital.

3.26a–d Prognosis in AMI

AMI is a medical emergency with a poor prognosis. Approximately 40% of all patients with AMI die either acutely or within a year of the attack. Up to one-half of these deaths occur before hospital admission as a result of Ventricular Failure (VF). After hospital admission, and in the next year, the major determinant of outcome is the severity of LV damage, patients with heart failure having a particularly poor prognosis.

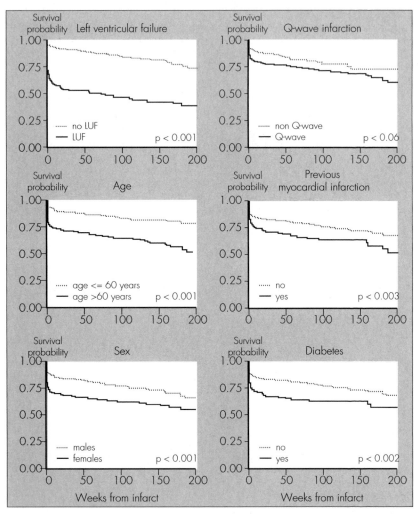

3.26a Prognosis in AMI according to baseline characteristics. These survival curves are for over 600 patients admitted to a coronary care unit. The data are stratified for major predictors of outcome. Note that patients with LV failure and patients aged over 60 have a particularly poor prognosis.

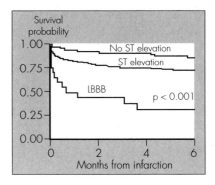

3.26b Prognosis in AMI according to the presenting ECG. These survival curves are for over 800 patients with AMI admitted to a coronary care unit. The presenting ECG is a powerful predictor of outcome, with risk increasing from a low level in patients without ST elevation, through an intermediate level in patients with ST elevation to a very high level in patients with left bundle branch block.

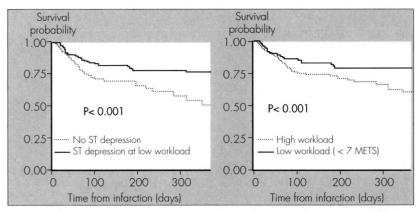

3.26c Prognosis in AMI: predischarge treadmill stress testing. These survival curves are for 256 patients who underwent predischarge treadmill stress testing. Note that patients who developed ST depression at low workload and patients unable to exercise to more than 7 mets have a significantly worse prognosis in the first year. Nevertheless, it must be recognized that in terms of diagnostic accuracy a predischarge treadmill stress test is of limited value for risk stratification.

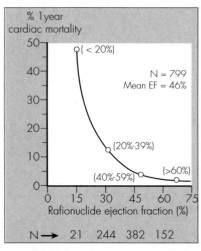

3.26d Prognosis in AMI: LV function. LV function is a powerful predictor of outcome. These data are for 799 patients with a recent myocardial infarction who underwent radionuclide ventriculography. Note the almost exponential relationship between LV function (measured as ejection fraction) and 1-year cardiac mortality, patients with an ejection fraction of less than 40% having a particularly poor prognosis.

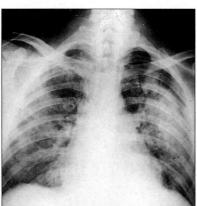

3.27 Complications of AMI: heart failure

Heart failure, as it reflects LV function, is the major determinant of prognosis in patients admitted to hospital with AMI. It is best diagnosed by the chest radiograph. In this example, the heart has not yet had time to enlarge but there is prominent alveolar pulmonary oedema in a perihilar distribution, giving a typical bat-wing appearance.

3.28a–d Complications of AMI: tachyarrhythmias

VF remains the major cause of death early after the onset of symptoms, before hospital admission. After admission, however, cardiac tachyarrhythmias can be treated and are rarely lethal.

Ventricular tachycardia is more sinister. n this example, sinus rhythm gives way to rapid ventricular tachycardia.

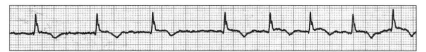

3.28a A trial fibrillation complicating AMI. AF is common in AMI but usually reverts spontaneously to sinus rhythm. This was an inferior infarct and the rate is rather slow.

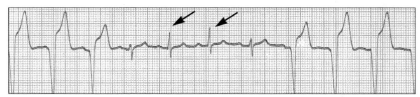

3.28b Accelerated idioventricular rhythm complicating AMI. Accelerated idioventricular rhythm is typically episodic, alternating with episodes of sinus rhythm. In this example, it is interrupted by 'fusion' beats (part sinus and part idio-ventricular in origin) and two sinus beats (arrowed).

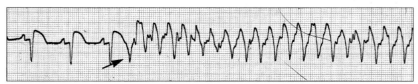

3.28c Ventricular tachycardia complicating AMI. A very early 'R on T' ectotic beat (arrowed) triggers rapid and life threatening ventricular tachycardia.

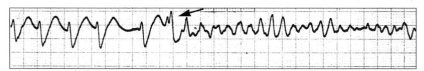

3.28d Ventricular fibrillation complicating AMI. Again, an early 'R on T' ectotic beat (arrowed) triggers a ventricular arrhythmia, this time ventricular fibrillation.

3.29a–c Complications of AMI: conduction defects and bradyarrhythmias in inferior myocardial infarction.

Bradyarrhythmias and conduction defects are very common in inferior myocardial infarction because of autonomic reflexes which tend to slow the sinus rate and delay AV conduction. Treatment with atropine is usually effective.

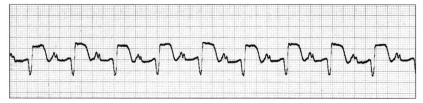

3.29a 1st degree AV block. Marked PR prolongation and ST elevation in acute inferior infarction.

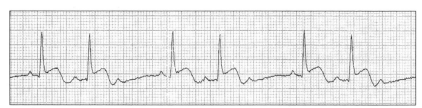

3.29b Type 1 AV block (Wenckebach). Three successive Wenckebach cycles are shown, each characterized by progressive PR prolongation until a beat is dropped. As the block is at nodal level, ventricular depolarization occurs by normal pathways, resulting in a narrow QRS complex.

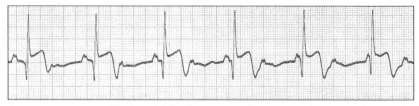

3.29c Complete AV block (nodal level). Dissociated P waves and QRS complexes with a junctional escape rhythm. As the block is at nodal level, ventricular depolarization occurs by normal pathways resulting in a narrow QRS complex.

3.30a–e Conduction defects and bradyarrhythmias in anterior myocardial infarction.

In contrast to inferior myocardial infarction which affects the conduction system indirectly (and temporarily) by autonomic effects on the AV node, anterior infarction affects AV conduction directly (and often permanently) by damaging the bundle branches.

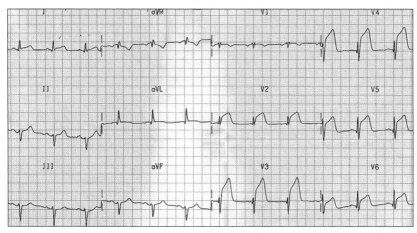

3.30a Left axis deviation ('left anterior hemiblock') complicating anterior infarction. The axis shift reflects damage to the anterior division of the left bundle and is a poor prognostic sign.

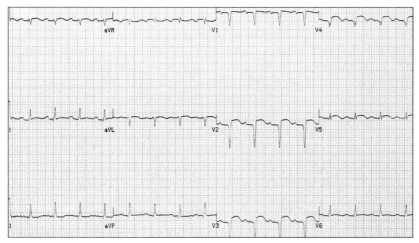

3.30b Right axis deviation ('left posterior hemiblock') complicating anterior infarction. The axis shift reflects damage to the posterior division of the left bundle and is a poor prognostic sign. Note also the prolongation of the PR interval (1st degree AV block).

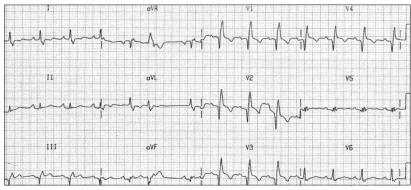

3.30c Right bundle branch block complicating anterior infarction. Right bundle branch block (broad QRS complex, late R wave in V1 and deep S waves in 1 and V6) is a poor prognostic sign.

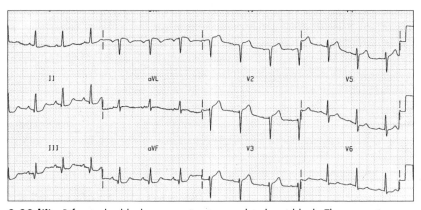

3.30d(i) Bifascicular block progressing to complete heart block. The presenting ECG shows evolving anterior infarction evidenced by ST elevation in leads V1 to V4. AV conduction is normal. .

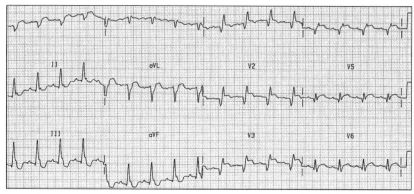

3.30d(ii) 6 hours later, the patient developed right bundle branch block and right axis deviation (bifascicular block). AV conduction is now dependent upon the anterior division of the left bundle.

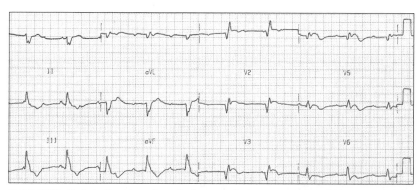

3.30d(iii) Only half an hour later, before prophylactic pacing could be instituted the block progressed to involve the anterior division of the left bundle resulting in complete heart block. This sequence of ECGs emphasizes the importance of prophylactic pacing when anterior myocardial infarction is complicated by bifascicular block.

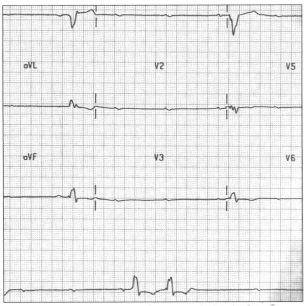

3.30e Mobitz type II block. The patient presented with extensive anterior myocardial infarction complicated by right bundle branch block and later became abruptly bradycardic because of intermittent failure of AV conduction. Note the nonconducted P waves in leads V1–V3. This demands emergency pacing.

3.31a–d Complications of myocardial infarction: myocardial rupture

Myocardial rupture may occur at any time during the course of AMI. It may involve the free wall of the left ventricle, when it is usually abruptly fatal or, alternatively, the interventricular septum or the papillary muscles, when survival is dependent on successful surgical repair.

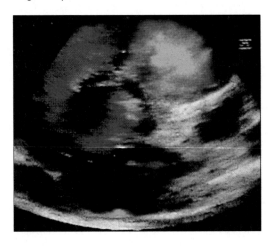

3.31a Ventricular septal defect: Doppler echocardiography. Ventricular septal defect may complicate anterior or inferior infarction. In this colour flow study, a large jet (coloured red) is seen flowing across an apically located ventricular septal defect. Treatment is by urgent surgical repair of the defect.

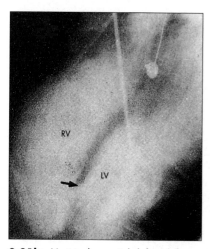

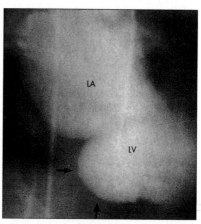

3.31b Ventricular septal defect: left ventriculogram. Note the prompt opacification of the right ventricle caused by the shunting of contrast through the ventricular septal defect (arrowed).

3.31c Papillary muscle rupture. This is a complication of inferior infarction. The left ventriculogram shows dense opacification of the left atrium caused by regurgitation through the incompetent mitral valve. The bulging dyskinetic inferior segment of the left ventricle (arrowed) is clearly visible. Treatment is by urgent mitral valve replacement.

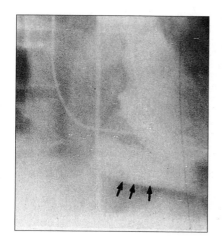

3.31d Free wall rupture. Rupture of the free wall of the left ventricle usually causes rapidly fatal tamponade. In this case, however, a false aneurysm has formed in the pericardial sac, protecting against tamponade. The left ventriculogram shows extravasation of contrast into the false aneurysm on the inferior surface of the heart. Treatment is by urgent surgical repair of the ruptured ventricle.

3.32a–c Complications of myocardial infarction: mural thrombus

Thrombus may develop on the endocardial wall of the left ventricle overlying infarcted myocardium. This predisposes to peripheral embolism.

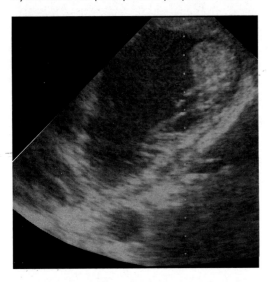

3.32a The echocardiogram (apical view) shows a large collection of thrombus at the apex of the left ventricle in a patient with recent anterior infarction.

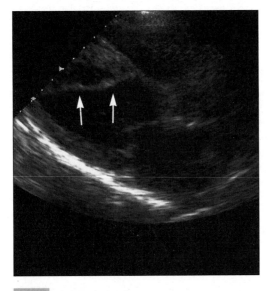

3.32b The echocardiogram (long axis view) shows a large collection of thrombus (arrowed), again in the cardiac apex, in a patient with recent anterior infarction.

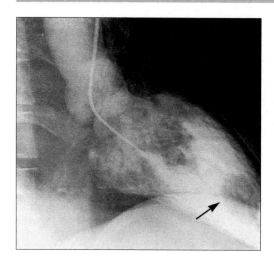

3.32c The left ventriculogram shows a large apical filling defect (arrowed) representing thrombus in a patient with recent anterior infarction.

3.33a–d Complications of AMI:
LV aneurysm

In approximately 10% of patients, the healing process after myocardial infarction is inadequate and a thin-walled ventricular aneurysm develops. This may be associated with persistent ST segment elevation on the ECG. The risk of rupture is negligible but in some patients the aneurysm can be a cause of cardiac arrhythmias, heart failure or clot embolization. Under these circumstances excision of the aneurysm may be required.

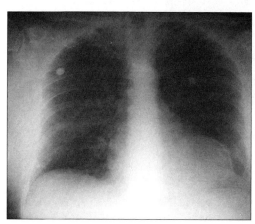

3.33a Chest radiograph: calcified LV aneurysm. A thin line of calcification is clearly visible along the LV wall. This appearance is caused by calcification in the wall of an aneurysm at the site of a previous infarct.

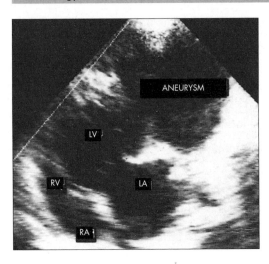

3.33b LV aneurysm: 2-D echocardiogram. A large 'blow out' of the LV wall occurred at the site marked with an arrow in this patient with anterior myocardial infarction. A large aneurysm developed, resulting in intractable heart failure which resolved after aneurysmectomy.

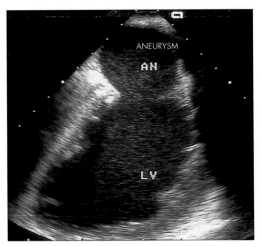

3.33c LV aneurysm: 2-D echocardiogram. As with the previous patient, a large aneurysmal sac developed after anterior myocardial infarction and required treatment by aneurysmectomy.

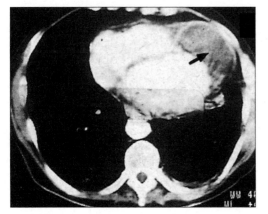

3.33d LV aneurysm: CT scan. This contrast-enhanced scan shows a large apical aneurysm (arrowed). It is filled with organized thrombus which has prevented penetration of contrast.

4.

Heart Failure

Classification of the aetiology of heart failure

Pathology	Phase of cardiac cycle affected		Ventricle affected	
	Systole	**Diastole**	**LV**	**RV**
Contractile dysfunction				
Ischaemic disease	++	+	++	+
Dilatated cardiomyopathy	++	–	++	+
Presssure overload				
Aortic stenosis	+	++	++	–
Hypertension	+	++	++	–
Pulmonary hypertension	+	++	–	++
Volume overload				
Aortic regurgitation	++	–	++	–
Mitral regurgitation	++	–	++	–
Atrial septal defect	++	–	–	++
Ventricular septal defect	++	–	++	+
Inadequate filling				
Hypertrophic cardiomyopathy	+	++	++	+
Restrictive cardiomyopathy	+	++	++	++
Constrictive pericarditis	–	++	+	++
Mitral stenosis	–	++	++	–
Tricuspid stenosis	–	++	–	++

4.1 The causes of heart failure

Coronary artery disease accounts for most cases of heart failure in this country but in developing countries rheumatic disease and cardiomyopathy remain more common. In this table, the causes of heart failure have been grouped according to its major pathophysiological determinants and an attempt has been made to identify the phase of the cardiac cycle (systole, diastole) and the ventricle (LV, RV) principally affected. Its classification is somewhat arbitrary, however, as many of the causes of heart failure affect both phases of the cardiac cycle and both ventricles.

4.2a–c Systolic heart failure

Systolic dysfunction predominates in ischaemic heart disease and dilated cardiomyopathy and plays an important role in heart failure caused by hypertrophic LV disease (hypertension, aortic stenosis, hypertrophic cardiomyopathy).

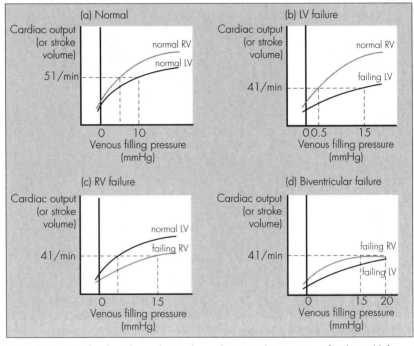

4.2a(i)–(iv) Pathophysiology: the Starling relation and integration of right and left ventricular function.

4.2a(i) In the normal heart, the resting cardiac output is produced by the right heart from a filling pressure of approximately 5 cm of water and by the left heart from a filling pressure of approximately 10 cm of water.

4.2a(ii) In left heart failure, the Starling curve of the left heart is depressed; to maintain cardiac output the filling pressure of the left heart is disproportionately raised and may lead to pulmonary venous congestion and even pulmonary oedema.

4.2a(iii) In right heart failure, the Starling curve of the right heart is depressed; the filling pressure of the right heart is disproportionately raised leading to elevated jugular venous pressure and dependent oedema.

4.2a(iv) In biventricular failure, both Starling curves are depressed and a normal cardiac output can only be achieved if both right and left-sided filling pressures are raised.

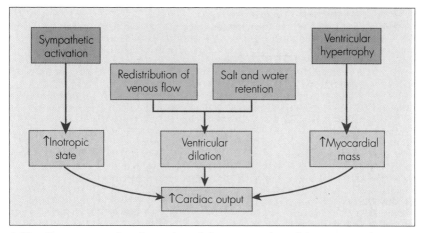

4.2b Compensatory physiology in heart failure. In acute heart failure, increased sympathetic activity is the only major mechanism available to support the heart; increasing inotropic drive and redistributing flow centrally, increases ventricular filling. If the patient survives this critical phase of decompensation, a new haemodynamic equilibrium may be established as the heart dilates and hypertrophies.

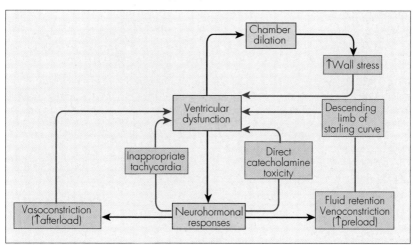

4.2c Vicious cycles of deterioration of systolic heart failure. A number of positive feedback cycles (in red) may contribute to the deterioration of heart failure. These are inter-related and may be regarded as a series of 'interlocking spirals'. It should be remembered that progression of the underlying aetiology of the heart failure is another potent cause of clinical deterioration.

4.3a–c Diastolic heart failure

In diastolic heart failure, there is an increased resistance to filling of one or both ventricles. The restrictive cardiomyopathy of amyloidosis is one of the clearest examples of impaired diastolic filling causing severe heart failure while systolic function is only slightly impaired. Impaired ventricular filling is also the major limitation to cardiac output in mitral and tricuspid stenosis and in constrictive pericarditis and acute tamponade. It also plays a major role in the heart failure associated with hypertrophic LV disease (e.g. hypertension, aortic stenosis, hypertrophic cardiomyopathy).

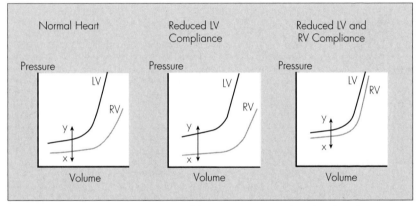

4.3a Pathophysiology of diastolic heart failure. Compliance describes the relation between pressure and volume and is the reciprocal of ventricular stiffness. During diastole both ventricles must fill to approximately the same volume.

Normal heart. The pressure, x, required to fill the thin-walled RV is considerably lower than the pressure, y, required to fill the thick-walled LV to the same volume. Thus, the RV compliance curve lies below the LV curve.

Reduced LV compliance (e.g. hypertrohpic disease). The LV is stiff and noncompliant. LV diastolic pressure, y, must rise considerably to maintain adequate filling and the LV compliance curve rises relative to the RV curve.

Reduced LV and RV compliance (constrictive pericarditis, restrictive cardiomyopathy). The diastolic filling of both ventricles is impeded equally. Thus, diastolic pressures of both ventricles (x and y) must rise and equilibrate to maintain adequate filling; the compliance curves, therefore, become almost superimposed.

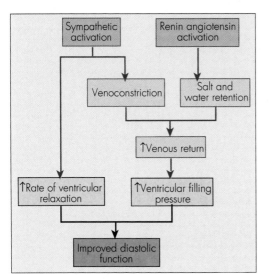

4.3b Compensatory physiology in diastolic heart failure. Activation of both the sympathetic nervous system and the renin–angiotensin mechanism improves diastolic function by the combined effect on ventricular filling pressure and ventricular relaxation.

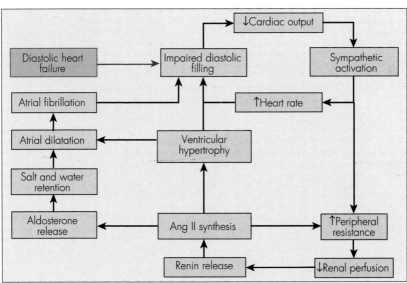

4.2c Vicious cycles of deterioration in diastolic heart failure. As heart failure worsens, increasing heart rate and ventricular hypertrophy, often accompanied by the development of atrial fibrillation, combine to aggravate the situation in a vicious cycle of deteriorating diastolic function.

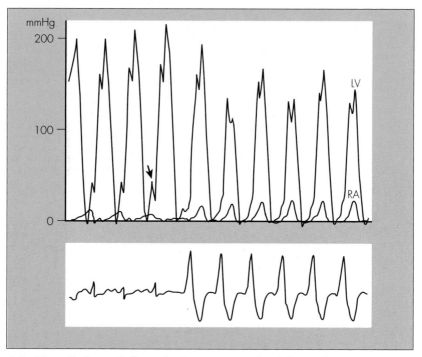

4.4 Diastolic heart failure: the importance of atrial systole

These are simultaneous recordings of the ECG and LV and RA pressure signals in hypertrophic cardiomyopathy. The first three complexes are sinus rhythm: note the prominent 'a' waves (arrowed) on the LV pressure signal reflecting vigorous atrial systole. Ventricular pacing after the 3rd complex produces a broad complex rhythm with AV dissociation. The loss of synchronized atrial contraction at end diastole impairs LV filling and causes abrupt deterioration in function shown by pulsus alternans, a fall in LV pressure and a rise in RA pressure. For this reason, atrial fibrillation is often poorly tolerated in hypertrophic cardiomyopathy and other causes of diastolic heart failure.

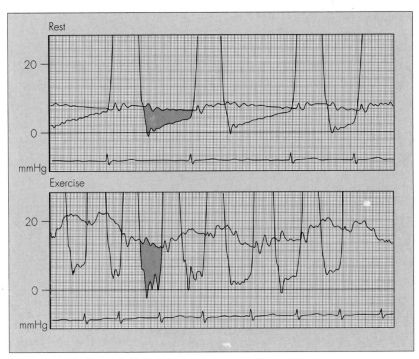

Rest

20

0

mmHg

Exercise

20

0

mmHg

4.5 Diastolic heart failure: the importance of heart rate

As heart rate increases, diastolic filling time shortens. This adversely affects all types of
diastolic heart failure, particularly mitral and tricuspid stenosis. In this example, LV and
pulmonary artery wedge (PAW) pressure signals are shown in mitral stenosis and atrial
fibrillation. The PAW pressure is a convenient measure of LA pressure obtained by right
heart catheterization using a balloon-tipped catheter (see 1.21). Under normal
circumstances, the PAW and LV pressures should be identical during diastole when the
mitral valve is open. In mitral stenosis, however, there is a gradient across the valve
and PAW pressure is higher than LV diastolic pressure. At rest (upper), the gradient
(shaded area) is trivial but during exercise (lower), tachycardia occurs and diastolic
filling is incomplete, resulting in a substantial increase in the gradient.

4.6a and b   Interaction of systolic and diastolic heart failure

In many patients with heart failure, an element of both systolic and diastolic dysfunction exists. This is particularly true in ischaemic disease and also in hypertrophic disease. These M-mode echocardiograms in two different patients with long-standing hypertension show concentric LV hypertrophy involving the inter ventricualr septum (IVS) and posterior wall (PW).

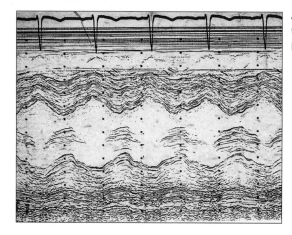

4.6a Contractile function of the hypertrophied LV is well preserved.

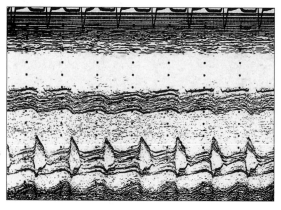

4.6b The ventricle has dilated and in addition to the diastolic dysfunction, there is now advanced systolic dysfunction with loss of contractile function.

4.7a–d Investigation of heart failure: chest radiograph

The chest radiograph provides a useful means of assessing heart size and pulmonary congestion in patients with heart failure. In most patients, the heart dilates as heart failure gets worse and LA pressure rises. Prominence of pulmonary veins (most marked in the upper lobes) is an early radiographic sign. As LA and pulmonary capillary pressures rise above 18 mmHg, transudation into the lung produces interstitial pulmonary oedema, characterized by prominence of the interlobular septa, most marked at the lung bases (Kerley B lines). Further rises in pressure lead to alveolar pulmonary oedema with air space consolidation, which is particularly prominent, in a perihilar ('bat-wing') distribution.

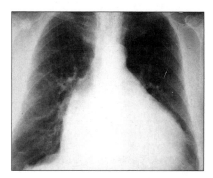

4.7a Heart failure: early pulmonary congestion. The heart is enlarged with prominent upper lobe pulmonary veins.

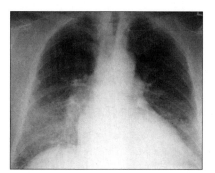

4.7b Heart failure: interstitial pulmonary oedema. The heart is enlarged with interstitial pulmonary oedema shown by Kerley B lines at the lung bases.

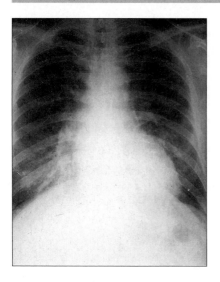

4.7c Heart failure: interstitial pulmonary oedema. As in the previous illustration, interstitial pulmonary oedema is clearly visible, but the heart is not enlarged. This patient has diastolic heart failure caused by amyloidosis.

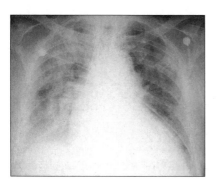

4.7d Heart failure: alveolar pulmonary oedema. Severe life-threatening pulmonary oedema shown by air space consolidation of both lung fields.

4.8a–d Investigation of heart failure: echocardiogram

The echocardiogram is potentially diagnostic of many of the cardiac defects that lead to heart failure. LV dilatation and *regional* contractile impairment indicate ischaemic disease, whereas four-chamber dilatation and *global* contractile impairment indicate dilated cardiomyopathy. Heart failure caused by valvular disease and tamponade can be readily diagnosed with an echocardiogram. Simultaneous Doppler studies permit identification of regurgitant jets through incompetent valves and shunting through septal defects.

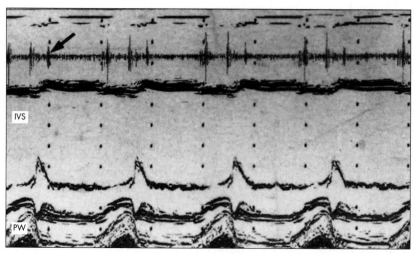

4.8a Heart failure: echocardiogram. This M-mode study shows considerable dilatation of the left ventricle. Note that the interventricular septum (IVS) is almost akinetic but the posterior wall (PW) is contracting normally. Regional contractile impairment of this type indicates coronary heart disease. The phonocardiogram, recorded simultaneously, shows normal 1st and 2nd heart sounds and also a 3rd heart sound (arrowed).

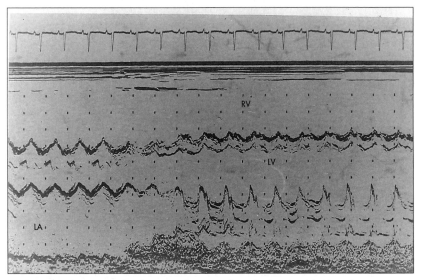

4.8b Heart failure: echocardiogram. This M-mode study shows a scan from the aortic root to the left ventricle (LV). Note that the left ventricle is severely dilated with global contractile impairment, indicating a cardiomyopathic process. Note also the considerable dilatation of the right ventricles (RV) located anteriorly and the left atrium (LA). Four-chamber dilatation of this type is typical of dilated cardiomyopathy.

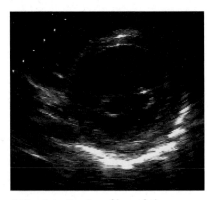

4.8c Investigation of heart failure: echocardiogram. This 2-D study (LV short axis view) shows a severely dilated ventricle typical of cardiomyopathy.

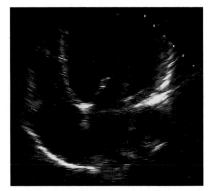

4.8d Investigation of heart failure: echocardiogram. This 2-D echo (LV four-chamber view) shows severe four-chamber dilatation typical of congestive cardiomyopathy.

4.9a and b Investigation of heart failure: radionuclide ventriculography

This provides an alternative 'noninvasive' way of examining LV cavity size and wall motion. It is particularly useful for quantifying ejection fraction and for identifying early ventricular impairment by application of provocative tests.

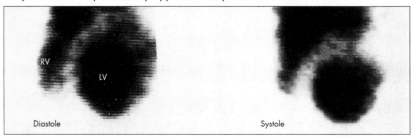

4.9a Radionuclide ventriculography: diastolic and systolic frames are shown in a patient with dilated cardiomyopathy. The LV cavity (arrowed) is severely dilated with global impairment of contractile function.

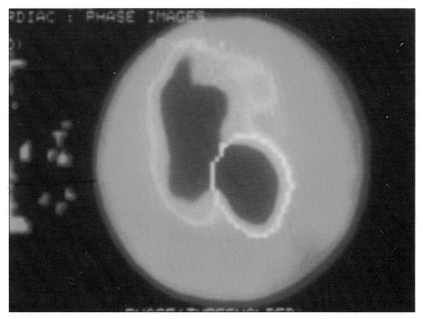

4.9b Radionuclide ventriculography: colour-coded study (diastolic frame) in dilated cardiomyopathy. The LV cavity dimension has been determined using computerized edge detection. The ventricle is severely dilated.

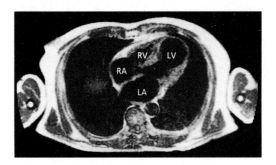

4.10 Investigation of heart failure: MRI scan
There is an aneurysm at the apex of the LV. Note the thin wall of the aneurysm compared with the normal thickness of the basal part of the ventricle.

4.11a–c   Investigation of heart failure: LV angiography
Angiography is not usually necessary for diagnostic purposes in heart failure because identical information can be obtained by noninvasive techniques, particularly echocardiography. Nevertheless, the majority of patients with heart failure have coronary artery disease and so cardiac catheterization is often performed to define the coronary anatomy. Angiographic images of the left ventricle can be obtained at the same study.

4.11a and b   LV angiography: diastolic and systolic frames.

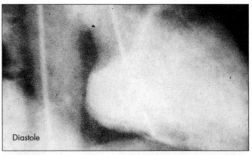

4.11a Diastole. The left ventricle is severely dilated.

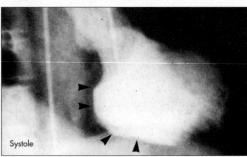

4.11b Systole. The systolic frame shows well preserved contraction of the anterior wall and apex but the infero-posterior wall (arrowed) is hypokinetic.Regional wall motion abnormality of this type points to coronary disease as the aetiology of heart failure.

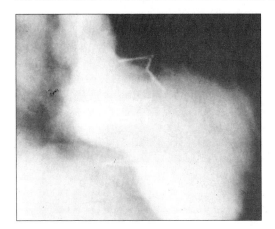

4.11c LV angiography: LV aneurysm. This systolic frame shows a large antero-apical aneurysm bulging during systole while the basal part of the ventricle contracts more normally. The patient had had coronary bypass surgery and had occluded the graft to the left anterior descending coronary artery.

4.12a and b Complications of heart failure

The major complications of heart failure are cardiac arrhythymias and sudden death. Other complications include intracardiac thrombus predisposing to peripheral embolism and stroke, and deep venous thrombosis predisposing to pulmonary embolism. Multi-organ failure characterizes the terminal stages of the disease.

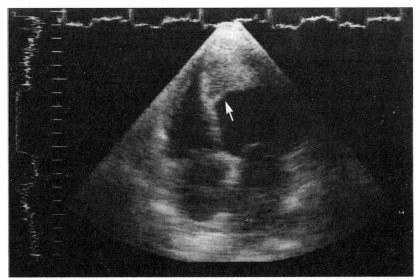

4.12a Complications of heart failure: left ventricular thrombus. The echocardiogram shows a dilated left ventricle with thrombus (arrowed) layered in the apex. This patient is at risk of systemic embolism and requires treatment with anticoagulants.

4.12b(i–iv) Cardiac arrhythmias. Atrial and ventricular arrhythmias occur commonly in heart failure. Atrial fibrillation (either paroxysmal or sustained) is probably the most common and like any arrhythmia may produce serious haemodynamic deterioration if the ventricular response is unduly rapid. Much more dangerous is ventricular tachycardia, which may herald sudden death in heart failure.

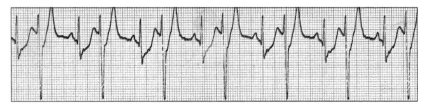

4.12b(i) Ectopic beats. These are a non-specific finding, but occur commonly in heart failure.

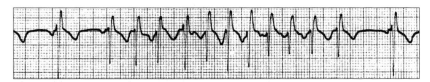

4.12b(ii) Paroxysmal Atrial fibrillation. AF is common in heart failure and may be paroxysmal (as in this example) or sustained.

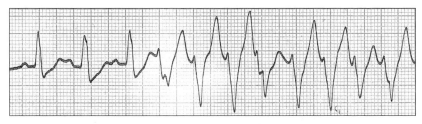

4.12b(iii) Ventricular tachycardia. VT occurs commonly in heart failure. In this example the rate is slow and is unlikely to provoke symptoms.

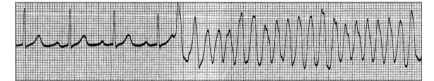

4.12b(iv) Ventricular tachycardia. Here the rate is rapid and life threatening.

4.13a and b   Prognosis in heart failure

Symptomatic heart failure rarely permits survival beyond 10 years. In patients who are severely symptomatic, the prognosis is still worse, with a 3 year mortality rate in excess of 50%.

Variables related to prognosis in chronic heart failure	
Severity of heart failure	NYHA grade
	Exercise capacity (especially peak $\dot{V}O_2$)
Aetiology of heart failure	CHF caused by coronary artery disease may be worse than CHF caused by cardiomyopathy
LV function/haemodynamics	Presence of 3rd heart sound
	Heart size on radiograph
	LV ejection fraction (or end systolic volume)
	Peak LV power output
Neurohormonal variables	Plasma noradrenaline
	Plasma Na^+ <137 mmol/l
	Hypomagnesaemia or hypermagnesaemia
ECG and arrythmyias	Left bundle branch block
	VT on 24 hr tape
	AF

4.13a   Variables related to prognosis in heart failure. Many different variables correlate with prognosis in heart failure. Advanced symptoms (measured by NYHA grade), reduced exercise capacity and reduced LV ejection fraction seem to be the most consistent predictors of poor survival.

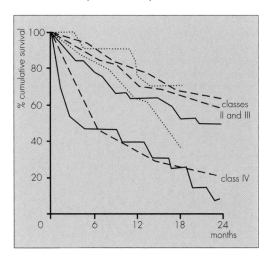

4.13b   Prognosis in heart failure related to NYHA class. Data from a number of different studies are shown. The 12-month mortality rate for NYHA class I failure is less than 10%, class II 10–20%, class III 30–50%, and class IV 30–70%.

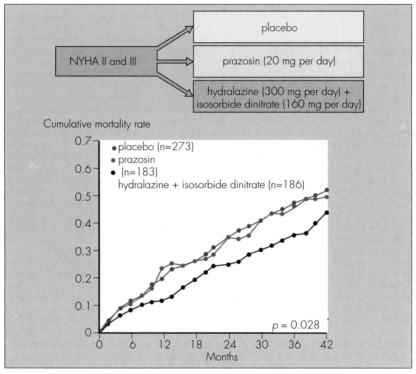

4.14 Effects of treatment on prognosis: vasodilators
The 1st Veterans Administration Co-operative Vasodilator Heart Failure Trial (VHeFT-1) randomized 642 patients with mild to moderate heart failure between placebo, prazosin and a combination of hydralazine and isosorbide dinitrate. The combination of hydralazine and isosorbide dinitrate lead to a 34% reduction in mortality over the next 2–4 years. Prazosin, on the other hand, was no better than placebo, probably because of the tachyphylaxis that occurs with this drug.

4.15a–c Effects of treatment on prognosis: angiotensin converting enzyme inhibitors

Angiotensin converting enzyme (ACE) inhibitors not only improve the symptoms of heart failure but also improve the long term survival.

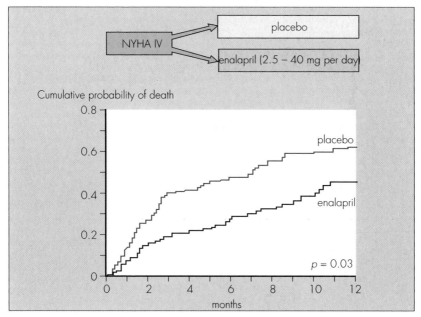

4.15a The Co-operative North Scandinavian Enalapril Survival Study (CONSENSUS). trial included patients with severe heart failure, all of whom were already being treated with diuretics, digoxin and in some cases , nitrates. The patients were randomized between enalapril and placebo as shown. Enalapril reduced mortality by 27% over the 1 year period.

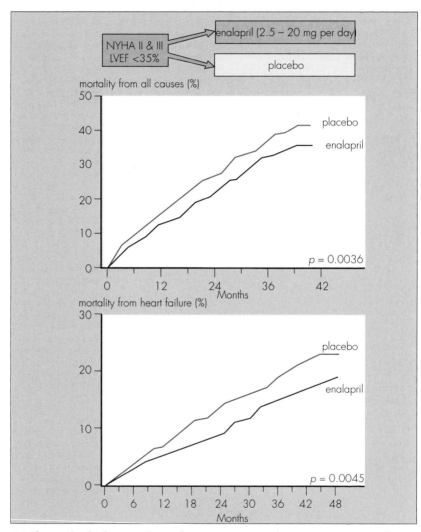

4.15b Study of Left Ventricular Dysfunction (SOLVD). In the SOLVD treatment trial, 2569 patients with moderately symptomatic heart failure were randomized between placebo or enalapril in addition to conventional therapy. Enalapril improved survival and reduced mortality over the 3–4 year follow-up period.

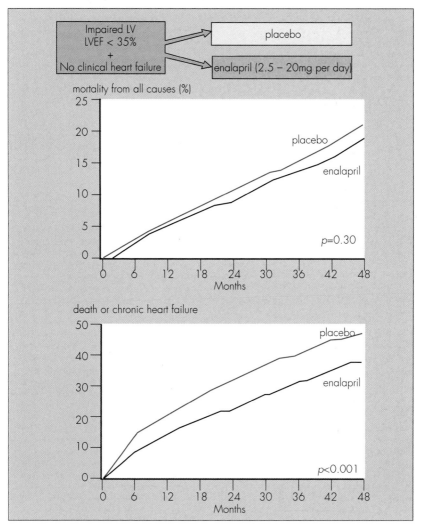

4.15c Study of Left Ventricular Dysfunction (SOLVD). In the prevention trial, 4228 patients with asymptomatic LV dysfunction were randomized between placebo and enalapril. Although the all cause mortality was unaffected, patients randomized to enalapril had a significantly reduced risk of developing heart failure or dying during the 48 month follow-up period.

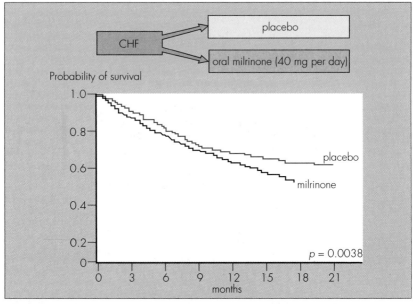

4.16 Effects of treatment on prognosis: inotropes

The only orally active inotrope licensed for clinical use in moderate to severe congestive heart failure is digoxin. The benefits of digoxin are well established in atrial fibrilation which occurs commonly in heart failure. For patients in sinus rhythm variable clinical benefit may occur but it has been less easy to show any prognostic improvement. Indeed, concern exists that inotropic drugs may have an adverse effect on prognosis as was recently shown in the Prospective Oral Milrinone Study (PROMISE). In this study, patients with severe chronic heart failure were randomized to receive oral milrinone (a phosphodiesterase inhibitor) or placebo in addition to standard heart failure treatment. Although some of the patients felt better on milrinone, it was associated with a 28% increase in mortality. The reasons for this are unclear.

4.17a–c Heart transplantation

In end stage heart failure, transplantation can produce a dramatic improvement in symptoms and prognosis. Undoubtedly the major limitation of this technique, however, is the lack of donor organs, which ensures that many patients referred for transplantation die on the waiting list before a suitable heart can be found. This problem will only be resolved when technology advances to allow use of animal donors or implantable mechanical devices.

Heart transplantation: selection guidelines

Selection guidelines	Relative contra-indications
Severe heart failure, refractory to medical treatment and not amenable to 'conventional' surgery (e.g. repair of congenital lesions, valve replacement)	Significant additional organic disease (e.g. active peptic ulcer, cancer)
	Pulmonary vascular resistance >6 Wood units
NYHA class IV symptoms	Peripheral or cerebrovascular disease
Age <60 years	Insulin requiring diabetes mellitus (?)
Expected survival > 1year	Psychiatric illness
Otherwise healthy, with well-preserved renal and liver function	
Compliant, well motivated	
Strong family support	

4.17a   Heart transplantation: selection guidelines.

Heart transplantation: complications

Complication	Management
Rejection (particularly first 2 months)	Pre-operative matching of donor ABO blood type
	Immunosuppression with cyclosporine, prednisolone, azathioprine or equine ATG
	Regular endomyocardial biopsy to reveal early histological signs of rejection
Infection (particularly first 2 months)	Antibiotic therapy at first sign
Accelerated artherosclerosis (after first year)	Correction of hypercholesterolaemia and other risk factors
Malignant lymphomas (after first year)	Radiation and cytotoxic therapy

4.17b   Heart transplantation: complications. The operative risk is small compared with the hazards of organ rejection. The risk of rejection is greatest within the first year of surgery but thereafter the threat of accelerated coronary atherosclerosis (the cause of which is unknown) becomes increasingly important.

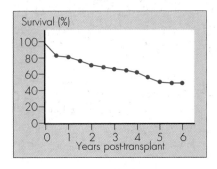

4.17c Heart transplantation: survival. For those patients who come to surgery the survival at 1 year is 80% falling to 60% after 6 years.

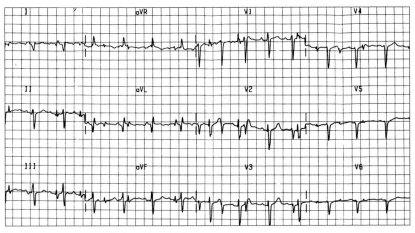

4.18 Heart transplantation: ECG

Heart transplantation involves excision of the diseased heart with preservation of the posterior atrial wall and suturing of the recipient atria to donor atria and great vessels to great vessels. The residual atrial tissue often generates a deflection on the surface ECG which is, of course, out of phase with the QRS complexes of the transplanted heart. An example is shown.

5.

Valvular Heart Disease

5.0 Valve Disease: Causes and Clinical Presentation

	Causes	Clinical presentation
Aortic stenosis	*Valve leaflet disease* Calcific disease – bicuspid valve Calcific disease – tricuspid valve Rheumatic disease	Dyspnoea Angina Syncope, LVF, sudden death
Aortic regurgitation	*Valve leaflet disease* Calcific disease – bicuspid valve Calcific disease – tricuspid valve Rheumatic disease Infective endocarditis* *Aortic root dilating disease* Marfan syndrome Hypertension Anklyosing spondylitis Aortic dissection*	Dyspnoea Angina LVF
Mitral stenosis	*Valve leaflet disease* Rheumatic disease Congenital disease (rare)	Dyspnoea, orthopnoea Haemoptysis AF (palpitation, embolism)
Mitral regugitation	*Valve leaflet disease* Prolapse Rheumatic disease Infective endocarditis* *Subvalvar disease* Chordal rupture* Papillary muscle dysfunction Papillary muscle rupture* *Dilating LV disease* LVF ('functional' MR)	Dyspnoea Orthopnoea AF (palpitation, embolism)
Pulmonary stenosis	*Valve leaflet disease* Congenital disease Rheumatic disease (rare)	Dyspnoea Systemic oedema
Pulmonary regugitation	*Valve leaflet disease* Infective endocarditis* (rare) *Pulmonary artery dilating disease* Pulmonary hypertension	Dyspnoea Systemic oedema
Tricuspid stenosis	*Valve leaflet disease* Rheumatic (rare)	Dyspnoea Systemic oedema
Tricuspid regugitation	*Valve leaflet disease* Infective endocarditis* Rheumatic *Dilating RV disease* RVF	Dyspnoea Systemic oedema

*These disorders produce acute valvular regurgitation

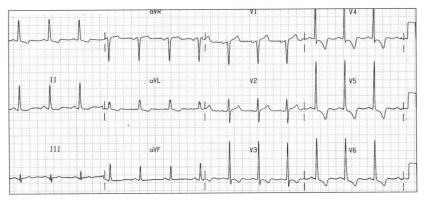

.5.2 Aortic stenosis: ECG

As aortic stenosis becomes more severe, compensatory LV hypertrophy produces exaggerated voltage deflections on the ECG, often associated with T wave inversion in the lateral leads. Voltage criteria for LV hypertrophy are fulfilled when the sum of the S and R wave deflections in leads V1 and V6, respectively, exceeds 35 mm (3.5 mV).

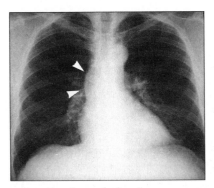

5.3a   Aortic stenosis: chest radiograph (postero-anterior projection). LV hypertrophy does not usually affect radiographic heart size which is usually normal in aortic stenosis. However, post-stenotic dilatation of the ascending aorta is often visible (arrowed).

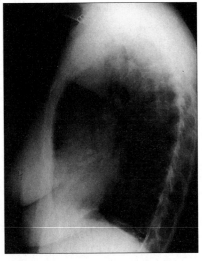

5.3b   Aortic stenosis: chest radiograph (lateral projection). Occasionally, the calcified valve is visible on the lateral film, as in this example.

5.4a–c Aortic stenosis: echocardiogram

Echocardiography is potentially diagnostic of nearly all the commonly occurring valve lesions. In aortic stenosis, a thickened, rigid valve can almost invariably be found.

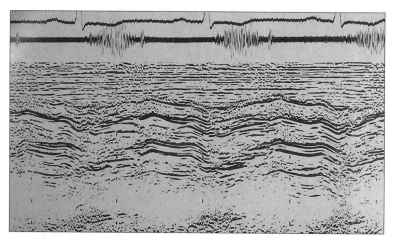

5.4a(i) Aortic stenosis: M-mode echocardiogram. A mass of dense echoes is visible in the aortic root caused by the densely calcified and rigid aortic valve.

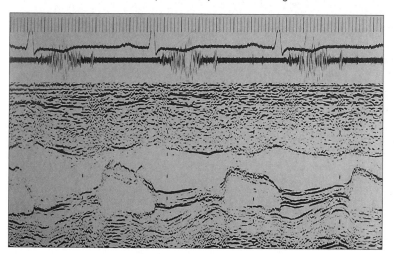

5.4a (ii) Scanning down to the left ventricle shows concentric hypertrophy involving the interventricular septum and posterior wall. Contractile function is well preserved. Note the ejection systolic murmur recorded on the phonocardiogram.

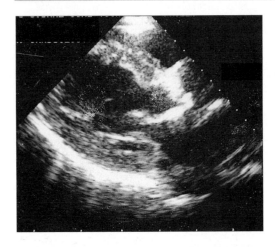

5.4b Aortic stenosis: 2-D echocardiogram (long axis view). The aortic valve is grossly thickened and highly echogenic. Concentric LV hypertrophy is present.

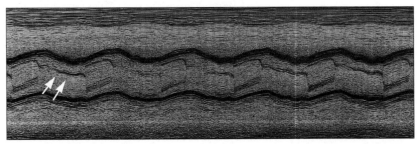

5.4c Bicuspid aortic valve: M-mode recording. The aortic valve appears normal and is probably not appreciably stenosed. However, the closure line of the valve leaflets during diastole (arrowed) lies eccentrically within the aortic root, which is typical of a congenitally diseased bicuspid valve. Turbulent flow across the abnormal valve leads to scarring and calcification of the leaflets in later life when the patient may present with symptoms of aortic stenosis (see also 11.7).

5.5a and b   Aortic stenosis: Doppler echocardiography

As valvular stenosis deteriorates, flow velocity across the valve increases because of a 'jet effect'. Doppler echocardiography permits quantitative assessment of flow velocity across the valve, from which the severity of stenosis can be calculated. Doppler technique is often preferred to cardiac catheterization for assessing the severity of stenotic valve lesions because it is noninvasive.

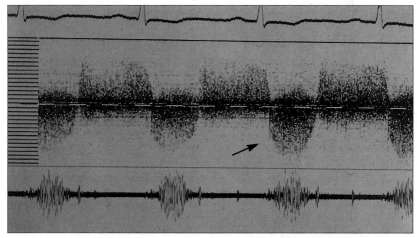

5.5a   Aortic stenosis: continuous wave Doppler. The aortic velocity signal (arrowed) is systolic in timing and coincides with the ejection murmur recorded on the phonocardiogram. Note the high-velocity diastolic flow in the opposite direction, indicating associated aortic regurgitation.

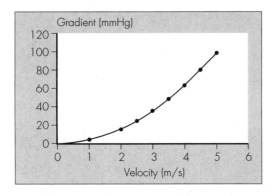

5.5b Aortic stenosis: derivation of pressure gradient from Doppler flow velocity. The graph defines the relationship between peak aortic flow velocity and the pressure gradient, derived from the modified Bernoulli equation (gradient = $4 \times velocity^2$).

5.6a–e Aortic stenosis: cardiac catheterization

Cardiac catheterization is rarely necessary for diagnostic purposes in valvular heart disease because it adds little to the information obtained noninvasively from Doppler echocardigraphy studies. Nevertheless, those patients with aortic stenosis (or other valve lesions) who are elderly and have angina need catheterization for coronary arteriography, which provides the opportunity to obtain haemodynamic data during the same study.

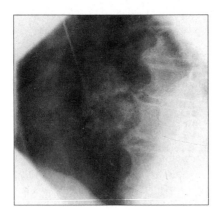

5.6a Aortic stenosis: fluoroscopy. The image intensifier in the catheter laboratory is considerably more sensitive than the routine chest radiograph for identifying intracardiac calcification. In this example, dense calcification of the aortic valve is clearly visible.

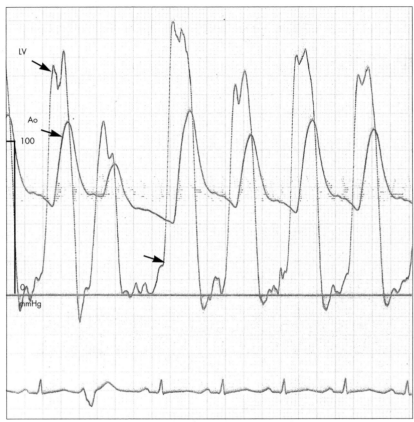

5.6b Aortic stenosis: simultaneous LV and Ao pressure signals. In the normal heart, the Ao and LV pressure signals should be superimposed throughout systole. Here, there is a peak systolic gradient of about 50 mmHg across the aortic valve. Note the prominent 'a' wave (arrowed), reflecting the major contribution that atrial systole makes to filling of the hypertrophied, noncompliant ventricle. Note also the pulsus alternans triggered by the extrasystole. Compare the minimal effect that the extrasystole has on the pressure gradient in aortic stenosis (fixed LV outflow obstruction) with the dramatic effect it has in hypertrophic cardiomyopathy (dynamic outflow obstruction: see 6.8b).

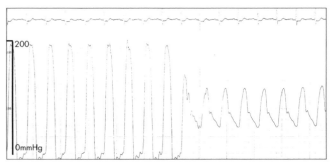

5.6c Aortic stenosis: pressure signals during catheter 'pullback' from left ventricle to aorta . In clinical practice, the peak systolic pressure gradient is calculated by pulling the catheter back from the left ventricle into the aorta across the diseased valve. The pullback recording shown here shows a pressure gradient of nearly 100 mmHg.

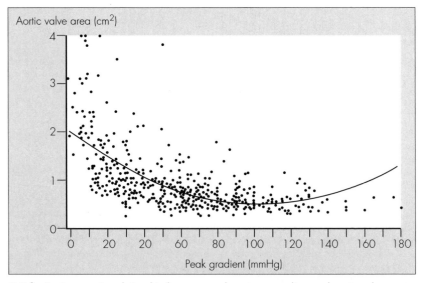

5.6d Aortic stenosis: relationship between peak pressure gradient and aortic valve area. This relationship is not linear because the peak systolic pressure gradient (see 5.5b and c) is dependent not only on the severity of the stenosis but also on the flow across the valve, patients with low cardiac output often have low pressure gradients even if the stenosis is severe. Generally, a peak systolic gradient > 50 mmHg reflects severe aortic stenosis (valve area less than 1 cm²) but when the gradient is lower, assessment of flow should always be taken into account before a final decision is made about stenosis severity.

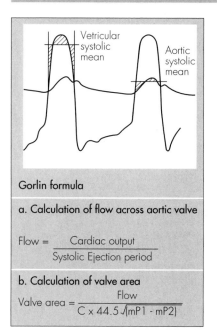

Gorlin formula

a. Calculation of flow across aortic valve

$$Flow = \frac{Cardiac\ output}{Systolic\ Ejection\ period}$$

b. Calculation of valve area

$$Valve\ area = \frac{Flow}{C \times 44.5 \sqrt{(mP1 - mP2)}}$$

5.6e Aortic stenosis: Gorlin formula for calculating valve area. Application of the formula, which takes into account the flow across the valve, provides a more accurate assessment of the severity of aortic stenosis. It requires measurement of the mean systolic gradient, a calculation of which is shown in the illustration. The flow is then calculated allowing valve area to be deduced in the manner shown. The Gorlin formula may also be applied for calculation of mitral valve area.

5.7a and b   Aortic stenosis: aortic balloon valvuloplasty

This catheter technique requires a balloon, introduced percutaneously, to be positioned across the aortic valve. Inflation of the balloon stretches the diseased valve and has been used to treat aortic stenosis. However, the procedure enjoyed only brief popularity and is no longer recommended because the risk is substantial and results are poor.

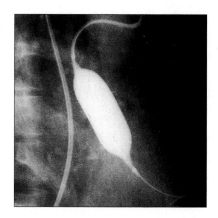

5.7a Aortic balloon valvuloplasty. A balloon is shown inflated across the aortic valve in a patient with severe aortic stenosis.

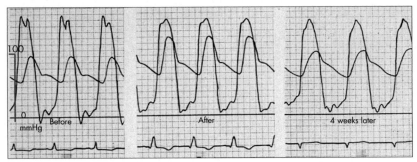

5.7b Aortic balloon valvuloplasty: haemodynamic result. Before valvuloplasty (left panel), a significant pressure gradient exists across the aortic valve. Immediately afterwards (middle panel), the pressure gradient is substantially reduced. However, 4 weeks later (right panel), the pressure gradient is as severe as it was before the procedure. This poor long term result is one of the main reasons why the procedure is no longer recommended.

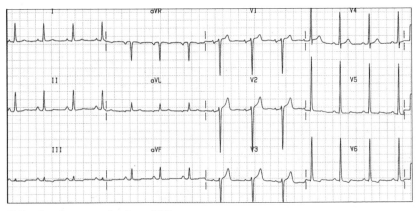

5.8 Aortic regurgitation: ECG

Aortic regurgitation volume loads the left ventricle which dilates and hypertrophies to produce exaggerated voltage deflections on the ECG.

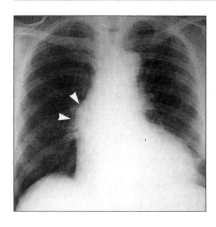

5.9 Aortic regurgitation: chest radiograph

The volume-loaded left ventricle dilates and produces enlargement of the cardiac silhouette. Note also the dilatation of the ascending aorta (arrowed) characteristic of this condition.

5.10a–f Aortic regurgitation: echocardiogram

The echocardiogram usually shows some dilatation of the ascending aorta and, in those patients with valve leaflet disease, abnormality of the valve itself. Variable LV dilatation and contractile dysfunction may also be seen.

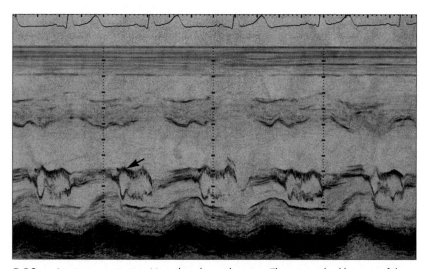

5.10a Aortic regurgitation: M-mode echocardiogram. There is early dilatation of the LV cavity but contractile function is well preserved. Note the fine vibrations on the anterior leaflet of the mitral valve (arrowed) caused by the regurgitant jet.

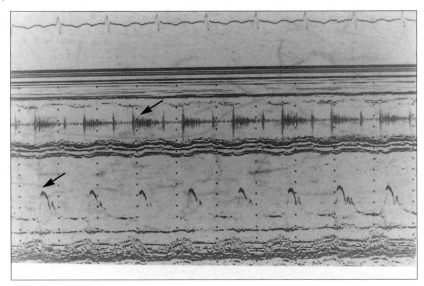

5.10b Aortic regurgitation: M-mode echocardiogram. There is severe LV dilatation and global contractile impairment. The fine vibrations on the anterior leaflet of the mitral valve (arrowed) are seen again. The phonocardiogram has recorded the early diastolic decrescendo murmur (arrowed). The prognosis here is poor but may have been better if aortic valve replacement earlier in the natural history of the disease had prevented deterioration in LV contractile function.

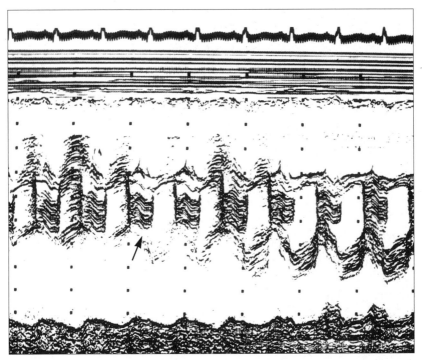

5.10c Aortic regurgitation: M mode echocardiogram. The patient contracted streptococcal endocarditis and presented with acute aortic regurgitation. Note the dense vegetations (arrowed) on the aortic valve.

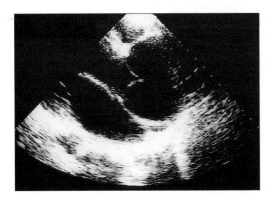

5.10d Aortic regurgitation: 2-D echocardiogram (long axis view). The patient had Marfan's syndrome. Note the aneurysmal dilatation of the aortic root, which has produced significant aortic regurgitation.

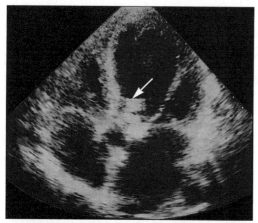

5.10e Aortic regurgitation: 2-D echocardiogram (four-chamber view). The patient acquired streptococcal endocarditis and presented with acute aortic regurgitation. Note the large vegetation (arrowed) adherent to the aortic valve leaflets.

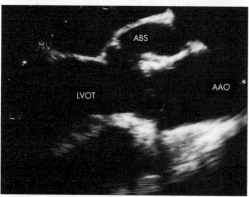

5.10f(i) Aortic regurgitation: transoesophageal echocardiograms. This patient presented with fever and signs of severe aortic regurgitation 6 months after aortic valve replacement (porcine zenograft). A paravalvular abscess (ABS) in the aortic root is shown communicating with the left ventricular outflow tract (LVOT) just below the aortic valve.

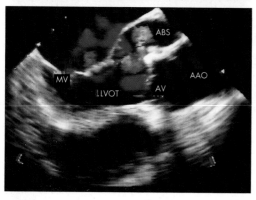

5.10f(ii). This colour flow Doppler study confirms free communication between the abscess cavity and the LVOT.

5.11a and b Aortic regurgitation: Doppler echocardiogram.

This provides a useful means of identifying the regurgitant jet and estimating its severity. Trivial, clinically unsuspected aortic regurgitation is seen commonly but, in the absence of symptoms or LV dilatation, rarely requires specific treatment.

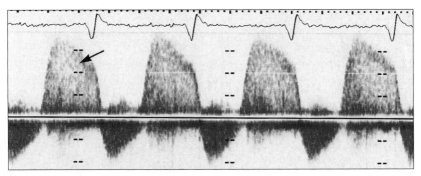

5.11a Aortic regurgitation: continuous wave Doppler. Note the high velocity jet of aortic regurgitation (arrowed) in early diastole. The velocity declines rapidly indicating haemodynamicaly significant aortic regurgitation.

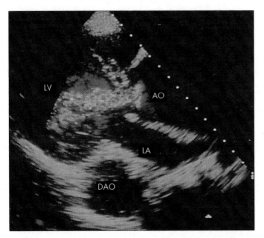

5.11b Aortic regurgitation: colour flow Doppler. This patient has an aneurysm involving the ascending (AO) and descending (DAO) aorta. There is a bright jet of aortic regurgitation extending beyond the anterior leaflet of the mitral valve towards the posterior wall of the left ventricle.

5.12a and b   Aortic regurgitation: aortic root angiogram

Angiography is rarely necessary for diagnostic purposes but in patients with aortic valve disease who require cardiac catheterization to rule out coronary artery disease, aortic root angiography is usually undertaken to provide additional information about the severity of regurgitation.

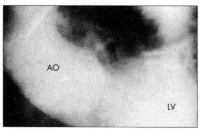

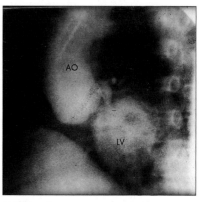

5.12a   Aortic regurgitation: aortic root angiogram. Contrast material has been injected into the ascending aorta through a catheter. Rapid opacification of the LV cavity has occurred because the aortic valve is incompetent. Note the dilatation of the proximal aorta, a typical finding in aortic valve disease.

5.12b   Aortic regurgitation: aortic root angiogram in acute aortic dissection. Dissection involving the ascending thoracic aorta may disrupt the aortic valve ring, causing acute aortic regurgitation.

5.13a and b   Mitral stenosis: electrocardiogram

ECG abnormalities commonly seen in mitral stenosis include atrial fibrillation and features of pulmonary hypertension. For those patients in sinus rhythm, evidence of LA enlargement is commonly present.

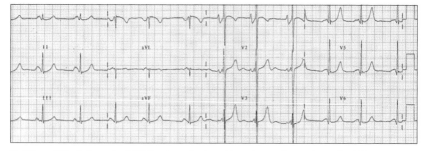

5.13a   Mitral stenosis: ECG in sinus rhythm. Note the prolonged, notched P wave, biphasic in lead V1, reflecting LA dilatation. This is commonly called 'P mitrale', although it may occur in any other disorder in which the left atrium is dilated.

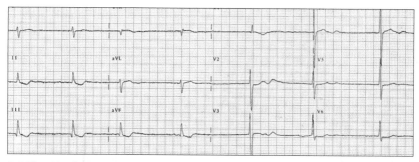

5.13b Mitral stenosis: ECG in patient with pulmonary hypertension. The rhythm is slow atrial fibrillation (AF). Features of RV hypertrophy include the prominent R wave in lead V1 and right axis deviation. The sagging ST segments are caused by digoxin but the slow ventricular rate indicates that the dose needs reducing.

5.14 a–d Mitral stenosis: chest radiograph

Mitral stenosis can often be diagnosed with confidence from the chest radiograph. Features of LA enlargement are invariably present. These include flattening or bulging of the left heart border below the main pulmonary artery (caused by leftwards displacement of the atrial appendage), widening of the carina (because of elevation of the left main bronchus), and the 'double density sign' at the right heart border (as a result of enlargement of the left atrium behind the right side of the heart). Mitral stenosis also produces signs of pulmonary congestion (see 4.6). Occasionally, calcification may be evident in the LA wall or in the mitral valve itself.

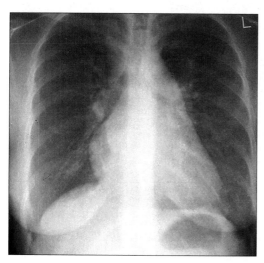

5.14a Mitral stenosis: chest radiograph (postero-anterior projection). Note the signs of LA enlargement: flattening of the left heart border, widening of the carina and the double density sign at the right heart border. Note also the prominent upper lobe pulmonary veins, reflecting raised LA pressure.

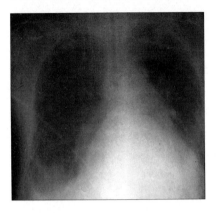

5.14b Mitral stenosis: chest radiograph (postero-anterior projection). Calcification is clearly visible in the wall of the left atrium. The patient had long-standing mitral valve disease with previous valve replacements.

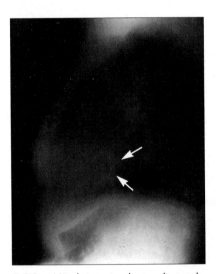

5.14c Mitral stenosis: chest radiograph (lateral projection). Mitral calcification as severe as this (arrowed) is unusual in mitral stenosis. The patient had chronic renal failure and was undergoing haemodialysis.

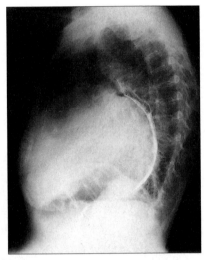

5.14d Mitral stenosis: barium swallow (lateral projection). This technique for demonstrating LA enlargement has been superseded by the echocardiogram but is occasionally undertaken in patients with advanced mitral stenosis who develop dysphagia. Note how the barium-filled oesophagus behind the heart is compressed against the posterior wall of the chest by the dilated left atrium.

5.15a–f Mitral stenosis: echocardiogram

The echocardiogram is diagnostic of rheumatic mitral valve disease. The thickened, rigid valve leaflets and the dilated left atrium can always be identified. As the pulmonary hypertension gets worse dilatation of the right-sided cardiac chambers also occurs.

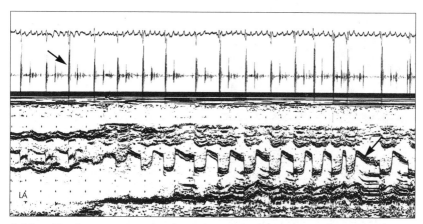

5.15a Mitral stenosis: M-mode echocardiogram. The mitral valve is thickened (arrowed) and the left atrium (LA), lying behind the aorta, is dilated. The ECG shows atrial fibrillation and the phonocardiogram shows a very loud 1st heart sound. The aortic valve (arrowed) is normal.

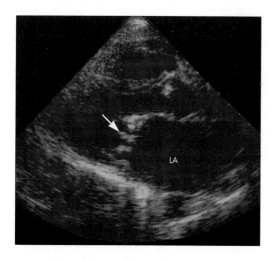

5.15b Mitral stenosis: 2-D echocardiogram (long axis view). Again, the mitral valve leaflets are densely thickened and the left atrium (LA) is severely dilated.

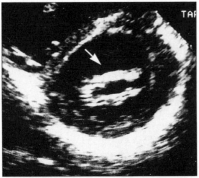

5.15c Mitral stenosis: 2-D echocardiogram (short axis view). The thickened mitral valve leaflets are clearly visible (arrowed). Separation of the valve leaflets in this diastolic frame is diminished, resulting in considerable reduction of the mitral valve area.

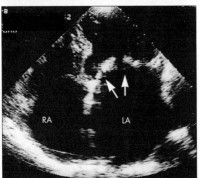

5.15d Mitral stenosis: 2-D echocardiogram (four-chamber view, diastolic frame). The thickened mitral valve leaflets (arrowed) are poorly separated, restricting flow across the valve. Raised pressure within the dilated left atrium (LA) has caused 'doming' of the mitral valve leaflets. Note also the dilated right-sided chambers caused by pulmonary hypertension.

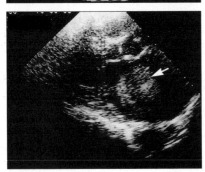

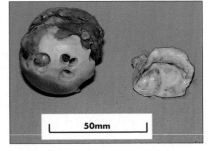

5.15e(i) Mitral stenosis: echocardiogram (2-D long axis view). A ball thrombus in the left atrium (arrowed), predisposing to peripheral embolism, is shown.

5.15e (ii) Surgical excision of the thrombus and the rheumatic mitral valve was undertaken.The surgical specimens, are shown here.

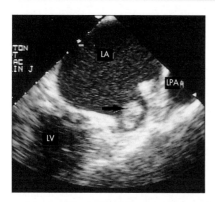

5.15f Mitral stenosis: transoesophageal echocardiogram. The left atrium (LA)is severely dilated and a large thrombus (arrowed) is visible in the appendage, emphasizing the importance of anticoagulation therapy in patients with mitral valve disease and atrial fibrillation.

5.16a and b Mitral stenosis: Doppler echocardiography

As valvular stenosis deteriorates, flow velocity across the valve increases as a result of a 'jet effect'. Doppler echocardiography permits quantitative assessment of flow velocity, from which the severity of stenosis can be calculated by application of the modified Bernoulli equation (gradient $= 4 \times velocity^2$).

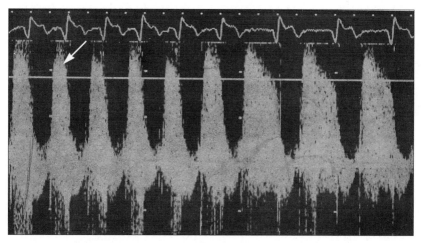

5.16a Mitral stenosis: continuous wave Doppler. The high-velocity diastolic jet across the mitral valve is arrowed. There is complete loss of the normal biphasic flow pattern because the patient is in atrial fibrillation. The peak velocity varies between 2 and 2.2 m/s, consistent with a gradient of 16–19 mmHg.

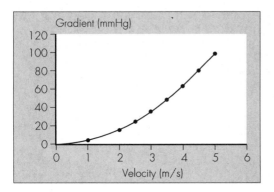

5.16b Mitral stenosis: Doppler echocardiography. This is a graphical representation of the relationship between the Doppler pressure half time (PHT) and calculated mitral valve area (MVA) derived from the relationship: MVA = 220/PHT

5.17a and b   Mitral stenosis: cardiac catheterization

Cardiac catheterization is no longer necessary for the diagnosis of mitral stenosis or assessment of its severity because Doppler echocardiography can provide identical information. Nevertheless, patients with mitral stenosis continue to have cardiac catheterization and the opportunity should always be taken to obtain simultaneous recordings of the pulmonary artery wedge pressure (an indirect measure of LA pressure; see 1.23) and the LV pressure. In the normal heart, the pressure signals should be effectively superimposed during diastole. In mitral stenosis, however, the LA pressure is higher than the LV diastolic pressure, the pressure gradient providing a measure of the severity of the mitral stenosis.

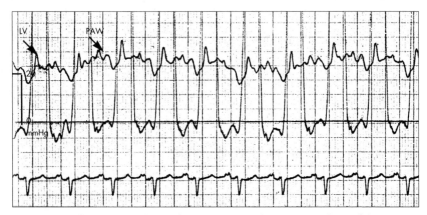

5.17a   Mitral stenosis: cardiac catheterization. Simultaneous recordings of the pulmonary artery wedge (PAW) and LV pressure signals are shown. Note that in diastole, there is a pressure gradient of about 15 mmHg indicating severe mitral stenosis. The ECG shows sinus rhythm with a typical broad P wave (P mitrale) reflecting LA enlargement.

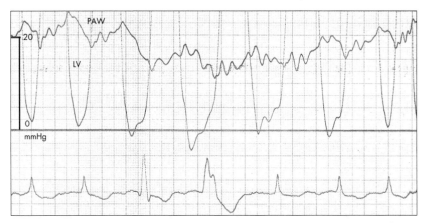

5.17b Mitral stenosis: cardiac catheterization. Again, simultaneous recordings of the PAW and LV pressure signals show a severe diastolic pressure gradient of between 10 and 18 mmHg. Note that the patient is in AF and the pressure gradient varies inversely with the RR interval, tending to increase as the RR interval shortens (see 4.4).

5.18a and b Mitral stenosis: balloon valvuloplasty

This technique may avoid the need for surgery in patients with mitral stenosis if the valve is noncalcified and competent. The balloon catheter is advanced from the femoral vein into the right atrium and then into the left atrium by trans-septal puncture. The balloon is positioned across the stenosed mitral valve and inflated. A good long term result can often be obtained, in contrast to aortic balloon valvuloplasty which is now no longer recommended (see 5.6c).

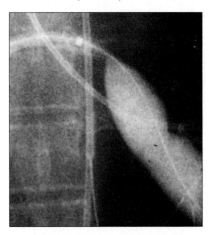

5.18a Mitral stenosis: balloon valvuloplasty. The balloon is shown inflated across the stenosed mitral valve. Note the 'waisted' central portion of the balloon where it is compressed in the valve orifice.

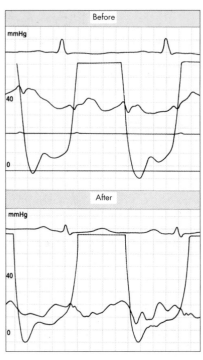

5.18b Mitral stenosis: balloon valvuloplasty. These are simultaneous recordings of the PAW and LV pressure signals before (top) and after (bottom) mitral valvuloplasty. Before the procedure, a substantial diastolic pressure gradient exists across the valve. Valvuloplasty has successfully reduced the gradient, almost to zero.

5.19a and b   Mitral regurgitation chest radiograph (postero-anterior projection)

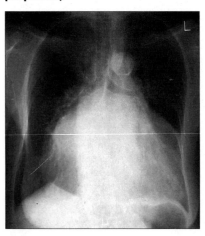

5.19a The penetrated film shows features of left atruim enlargement. Including widening of the carinal angle and a double density sign at the right heart border. The cardiac silhouette is considerably enlarged because the volume loaded left sided chambers are both severely dilated.

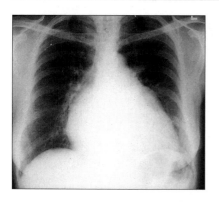

5.19b In this less penetrated film, the dilated upper lobe pulmonary veins are seen. Note also the flattened left heart border reflecting advanced left atrial dilitation.

5.20a–c Mitral regurgitation: echocardiogram

The echocardiogram may show an abnormal mitral valve but in cases of 'subvalvular' mitral regurgitation caused by chordal or papillary muscle disease, the valve may appear normal. The volume-loaded left ventricle tends to dilate and often shows vigorous systolic contraction early in the natural history of the disease. If valve replacement is delayed, progressive LV dilatation and contractile failure develop.

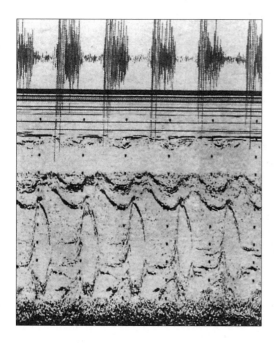

5.20a Mitral regurgitation: M-mode echocardiogram. The patient presented with symptoms of severe mitral regurgitation caused by chordal rupture. Note the wide excursion of the mitral valve leaflets during diastole and the vigorous contraction of the somewhat dilated left ventricle. The systolic murmur has been simultaneously recorded on the phonocardiogram.

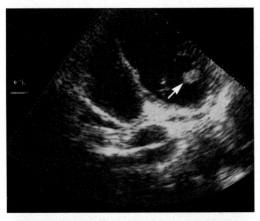

5.20b Mitral regurgitation: 2-D echocardiogram (apical four-chamber view). The patient had streptococcal endocarditis. A large vegetation (arrowed) is adherent to the posterior leaflet of the mitral valve.

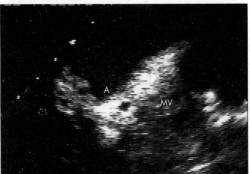

5.20c(i) Mitral regurgitation: transoesophageal echocardiogram. The patient had streptococcal endocarditis and a large mitral valve abscess. There is a large vegetation on the mitral valve (MV) in association with an abscess (A).

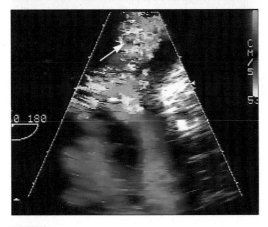

5.20c(ii) The colour flow Doppler study shows a large jet of mitral regurgitation involving much of the LA cavity.

5.21a and b   Mitral regurgitation: Doppler echocardiography

This provides a useful means of identifying the regurgitant jet and estimating its severity. Trivial, clinically unsuspected mitral regurgitation is seen commonly but, in the absence of symptoms or LV dilatation, rarely requires specific treatment.

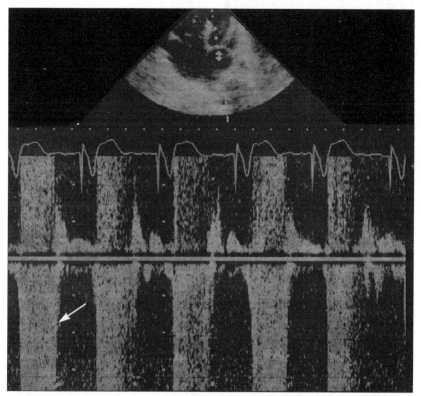

5.21a   Mitral regurgitation: pulsed Doppler. A range-gating facility permits frequency sampling from any point within the heart, preselected on the echocardiogram. Here, frequency sampling from the left atrium (arrowed on echocardiogram) has identified a large systolic jet (arrowed) in a patient with severe mitral regurgitation.

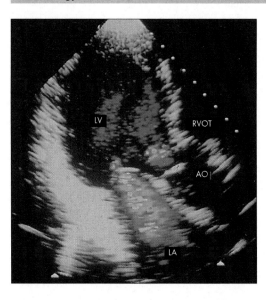

5.21b Mitral regurgitation: colour flow Doppler. This is an apical long axis view of the heart showing a large jet of mitral regurgitation (blue) occupying most of the LA cavity.

5.22a and b   Mitral regurgitation: cardiac catheterization

The severity of mitral regurgitation can be assessed by left ventriculography, although this does not provide information that cannot be obtained noninvasively by Doppler echocardiography. During cardiac catheterization, a haemodynamic assessment can also be made by measuring PA and PAW pressures.

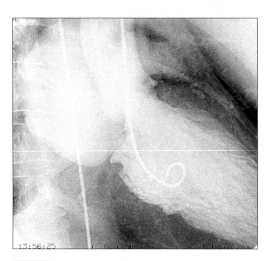

5.22a Mitral regurgitation: cardiac catheterization (left ventriculogram). Contrast injection into the left ventricle has resulted in prompt opacification of the left atrium owing to back flow across the diseased mitral valve.

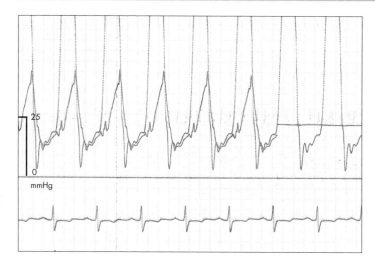

5.22b Mitral regurgitation: cardiac catheterization (haemodynamic assessment). Simultaneous recordings of the PAW and LV pressure signals are shown in acute mitral regurgitation caused by chordal rupture. LV diastolic pressure is elevated (about 20 mmHg) but there is no pressure gradient across the mitral valve. Note the large systolic 'v' wave on the PAW trace reflecting the surge in LA pressure caused by regurgitation through the mitral valve. The 'v' wave may be less prominent in chronic mitral regurgitation as the left atrium dilates and becomes more compliant.

5.23a–c Mitral valve prolapse

This is a common and usually asymptomatic condition in which one or both of the mitral valve leaflets bulge back into the left atrium during systole. This may produce trivial mitral regurgitation in some cases but only rarely is it severe. Mitral valve prolapse affects about 5% of the population and is particularly common in young women. The cause is unknown but it may be associated with a variety of cardiac and systemic disorders. Most cases, however, are idiopathic and are characterized by myxomatous degeneration of the valve leaflet tissue. Typically, a mid-systolic click is followed by a murmur. The echocardiogram is diagnostic.

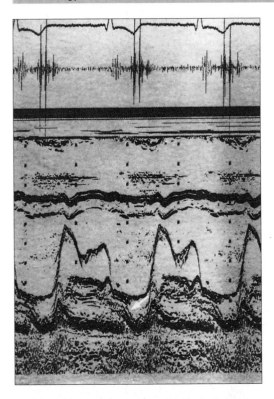

5.23a Mitral valve prolapse: M-mode echocardiogram. Systolic prolapse of the posterior mitral valve leaflet is shown (arrowed). The click and murmur have been recorded on the phonocardiogram. In this case two additional clicks of greater intensity occur later in systole.

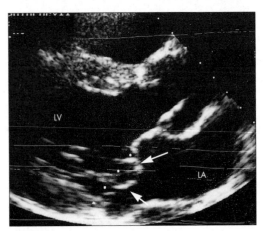

5.23b Mitral valve prolapse: 2-D echocardiogram (long axis view). This is a systolic frame (aortic valve open). The mitral valve plane is defined by the white dots. Note how the anterior and posterior leaflets of the mitral valve are bulging backwards behind the valve (arrowed) plane (denoted by the white dots) into the left atrium (LA).

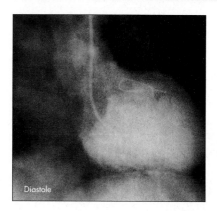

5.23c(i) Mitral valve prolapse: left ventriculograms. In diastole the left ventricle is dilated. Because of previous myocardial infarction. (Note sternal sutures from previous CABG).

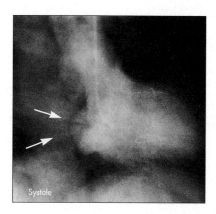

5.23c(ii) The systolic frame shows the two leaflets of the mitral valve (arrowed) bulging backwards into the left atrium.

5.24a–f Valve surgery

Surgery has revolutionized the management of valvular heart disease and can produce complete haemodynamic correction. The timing of valve surgery is important. If it is delayed until ventricular dysfunction or pulmonary hypertension have become irreversible, the risks are greater and the results less satisfactory. In mitral stenosis, dilatation of the valve (valvotomy) is effective if the valve is competent and not calcified (see 5.16). Regurgitation through the AV valves can sometimes be corrected by repair procedures. In most cases of valvular heart disease, however, surgical correction requires replacement of the valve with a tissue graft or a prosthesis.

5.24a   Valve surgery: indications for valve replacement. Indications for valve replacement are arrayed around a cine frame showing a coronary arteriogram with a ball-and-cage prosthesis in the mitral position and a porcine xenograft in the aortic position. Indications for surgery in aortic and mitral stenosis are well defined but in aortic and mitral regurgitation they are less clear cut. It is vital, however, that surgery is timed to prevent irreversible deterioration of LV contractile function.

Mitral valve replacement
Mitral stenosis
• Dyspnoea not controlled by diuretics
• Pulmonary hypertension and RV failure

Aortic valve replacement
Aortic Stenosis
• Any symptoms
• Systolic gradient>50mmHg
• Systolic gradient<50mmHg if LV function impaired

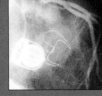

Mitral valve replacement
Mitral regurgitation
• Dyspnoea not controlled by diuretics

• Worsening LV dilatation and contractile failure.

Aortic valve replacement
Aortic regurgitation
• Dyspnoea not controlled by diuretics

• Worsening LV dilatation and contractile failure

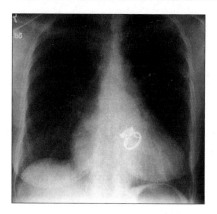

5.24b Valve surgery: chest radiograph (postero-anterior projection). Two tilting disc prosthetic valves are visible (presumably aortic and mitral) but it is difficult to be sure which is which in this projection.

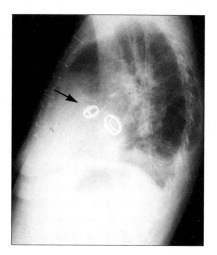

5.24c Valve surgery: chest radiograph (lateral projection). This projection permits confident identification of the valves: the aortic valve (arrowed) lies anterior to the mitral valve.

5.24d(i) and (ii) Valve surgery: 2-D echocardiogram and colour flow Doppler.

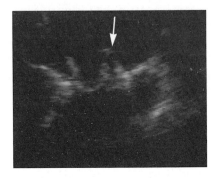

5.24d (i) A porcine xenograft is shown in the mitral position. The stent in which the valve is mounted is clearly visible (arrowed).

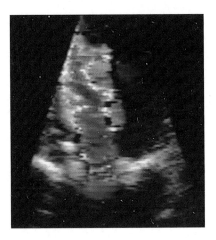

5.24d (ii) The valve is functioning normally and the Doppler study confirms normal forward flow through the xenograft in diastole.

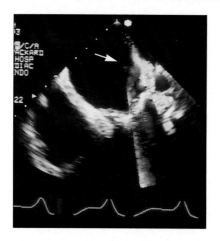

5.24e Valve surgery: paraprosthetic leak. This transoesophageal echocardiogram shows a prosthetic valve in the mitral position. The colour flow Doppler study shows a localized paraprosthetic leak with a regurgitant jet (arrowed) directed into the left atrium.

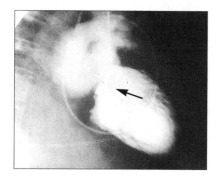

5.24f Valve surgery: left ventriculogram. Mitral valve replacement (the prosthesis is arrowed) was complicated by endocarditis with a paraprosthetic defect. Note how contrast injection into the left ventricle has resulted in (prompt) opacification of the left atrium owing to back flow through the defect.

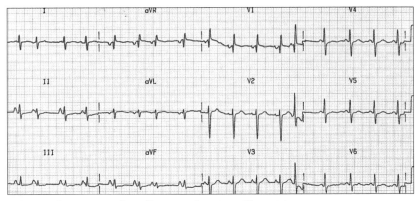

5.25 Pulmonary valve disease: electrocardiogram

RV hypertrophy and RA enlargement are shown by the prominent R wave in lead V1 and the tall P waves (P pulmonale) in the inferior limb leads, respectively. The changes are nonspecific and may also occur in pulmonary hypertension.

5.26a and b Pulmonary valve disease: chest radiograph

Dilatation of the main pulmonary artery is almost invariable in clinically significant pulmonary valve disease.

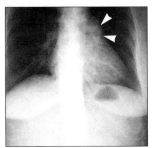

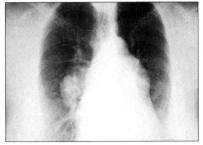

5.26a Pulmonary stenosis: chest radiograph projection. Note the poststenotic dilatation of the pulmonary artery (PA) (arrowed). In most cases, no treatment is necessary but in severe pulmonary stenosis surgical correction is required. Balloon valvuloplasty has largely replaced surgery for the treatment of pulmonary stenosis in infants.

5.26b Pulmonary regurgitation: chest radiograph (PA projection). Pulmonary hypertension is the usual cause of pulmonary regurgitation. This patient had Eisenmenger syndrome with severe pulmonary hypertension, reflected by the oligaemic lung films and the gross dilatation of the proximal pulmonary arteries. Pulmonary regurgitation is essentially a functional phenomenon in these patients and makes only a minor contribution to the haemodynamic derangement.

5.27a and b Pulmonary valve disease: echo-Doppler studies

Although the pulmonary valve may be difficult to image by transthoracic echocardiography, in most patients abnormalities of the valve can be detected by skilled operators. Doppler studies permit quantitative assessment of the severity of pulmonary stenosis and also identification of pulmonary regurgitation.

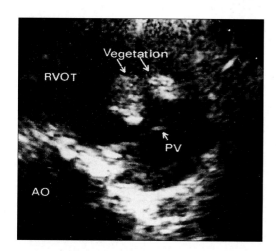

5.27a Pulmonary valve disease: 2-D echocardiogram. Infective endocarditis of the pulmonary and tricuspid valves is unusual and occurs most commonly in individuals who intravenously abuse drugs or who are immunocompromised. Here, large vegetations caused by fungal endocarditis are shown on the PV.

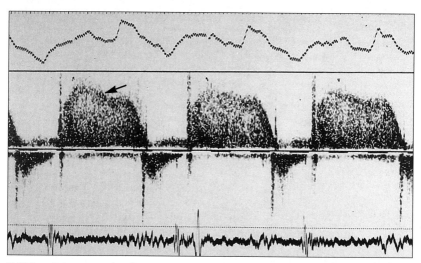

5.27b Pulmonary valve disease: continuous wave Doppler. The diastolic jet of pulmonary regurgitation (arrowed) is shown in a patient with advanced pulmonary hypertension.

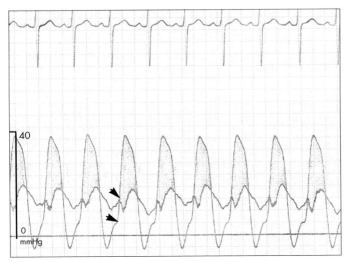

5.28 Pulmonary stenosis: cardiac catheterization

Simultaneous recordings of the RV and PAW pressure signals are shown. Note the systolic gradient of about 50 mmHg reflecting moderately severe pulmonary stenosis. Note also the prominent 'a' waves (arrowed) on the pulmonary artery and RV pressure signals reflecting the vigorous RA systole required to fill the hypertrophied noncompliant right ventricle.

5.29a and b Tricuspid valve disease

The most common tricuspid valve lesion is 'functional' regurgitation caused by stretching of the valve ring in patients with pulmonary hypertension and RV failure. Primary disease (rheumatic, carcinoid, endocarditis) of the tricuspid valve is rare.

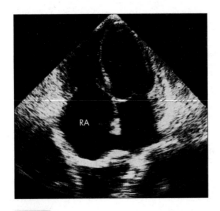

5.29a Tricuspid valve disease: 2-D echocardiogram. The patient had carcinoid syndrome with hepatic metastases and tricuspid regurgitation. This is a systolic frame: the mitral valve is closed but the damaged tricuspid valve leaflets are tethered and remain widely separated allowing free tricuspid regurgitation. The right atrium (RA) is severely dilated.

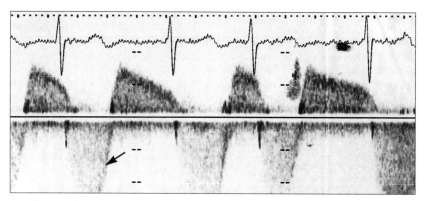

5.29b(i) and (ii) Tricuspid valve disease: continuous wave Doppler echocardiography. A prominent systolic jet (arrowed) is shown, reflecting severe tricuspid regurgitation. The patient also had tricuspid stenosis shown by the exaggerated diastolic flow velocity and the end diastolic velocity gradient.

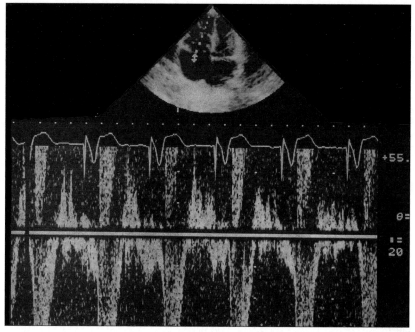

5.29b(ii) Tricuspid valve disease: pulsed wave Doppler. Sampling from right atrium (see 2-D echo) reveals a jet of tricuspid regurgitation (arrowed).

5.30a and b   Tricuspid valve disease: cardiac catheterization

Cardiac catheterization is of little diagnostic value in tricuspid valve disease. Tricuspid stenosis is difficult to assess and although tricuspid regurgitation produces a prominent systolic 'v' wave on the RA pressure signal, simple observation of the jugular venous pulse provides identical information (see 2.7a–e).

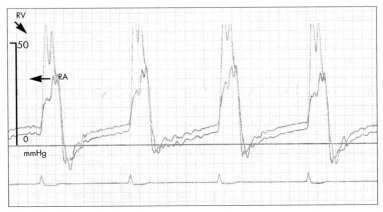

5.30a   Tricuspid regurgitation: haemodynamic assessment. Simultaneous recordings of the RA and RV pressure signals are shown. Note that during systole there is a sharp rise in RA pressure (giant 'v' wave) caused by the regurgitant jet.

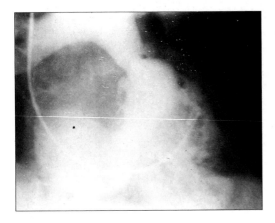

5.30b   Tricuspid regurgitation: right ventriculogram. Tricuspid regurgitation is best diagnosed by observation of the jugular venous pulse which shows a giant 'v' wave (see 5.30a). In this patient with carcinoid syndrome, RV angiograph was performed, which shows prompt opacification of the right atrium (RA) caused by free regurgitation of contrast through the tricuspid valve.

6.

Myocardial Disease

Cardiomyopathy

Chronic heart muscle disorder, unrelated to coronary disease,
valvular disease or hypertension

Cardiomyopathy: classification, pathophysiology and aetiology

Classification	Pathophysiology	Aetiology
Dilated cardiomyopathy	Ventricular dilatation and hypertrophy with global impairment of systolic contraction	Idiopathic, familial, viral alcoholism, doxorubicin toxicity, muscular dystrophy, pregnancy, puerperium
Hypertrophic cardiomyopathy	Ventricular hypertrophy with global impairment of diastolic relaxation	Idiopathic Familial
Restrictive cardiomyopathy	Global impairment of diastolic relaxation	Endomyocardial fibrosis (Loeffler's syndrome), amyloidosis, haemochromatosis

6.1 Cardiomyopathy: classification, pathophysiology and aetiology

Many, perhaps all, cases of hypertrophic cardiomyopathy are genetically determined. There may also be a genetic component to some cases of dilated cardiomyopathy, although occult viral infection is likely to be the more important underlying cause in many of the so-called idiopathic cases. Restrictive cardiomyopathy is common in the tropics, where endomyocardial fibrosis is the usual cause. In the UK, restrictive cardiomyopathy is more rare and is usually caused by amyloidosis.

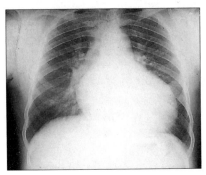

6.2 Dilated cardiomyopathy: chest radiograph

This chest radiograph shows a large heart and congested lung fields with prominent upper lobe pulmonary veins. The cardiothoracic ratio exceeds 0.55 suggesting dilatation of one or more chambers; although pericardial effusion can not be excluded.

6.3a–d Dilated cardiomyopathy: echocardiogram

The echocardiogram is usually diagnostic of dilated cardiomyopathy, showing LV dilatation and global contractile failure in the absence of valvular abnormalities. Commonly, all four cardiac chambers are dilated. Regional wall motion is most easily appreciated on dynamic 2-D images. Static images, on the other hand, such as those illustrating this book, do not permit wall motion analysis unless M-mode images are used.

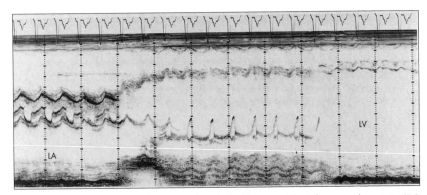

6.3a Dilated cardiomyopathy: M-mode echocardiogram. The left ventricular cavity (LV) is greatly dilated and global contractile failure is shown by the markedly reduced amplitude of both septal and posterior wall motion. The left atrium (LA) is also dilated but the aortic and mitral valves are normal.

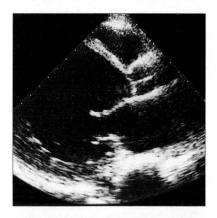

6.3b Dilated cardiomyopathy: 2-D echocardiogram (long axis view). The left ventricle is severely dilated and on the real–time recording, contractile function was severely diminished.

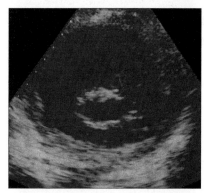

6.3c Dilated cardiomyopathy: 2-D echocardiogram (short axis view). Again, the left ventricle is severely dilated. This view is particularly useful for examining circumferential left ventricular shortening and showing regional abnormalities.

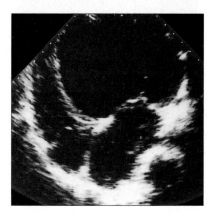

6.3d Dilated cardiomyopathy: 2-D echocardiogram (apical four-chamber view). The left ventricle is greatly dilated. This view is particularly useful for assessing the dimensions of all four cardiac chambers.

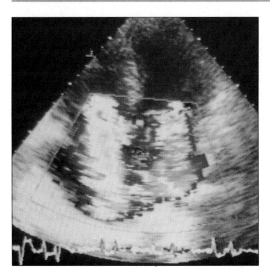

6.4 Dilated cardiomyopathy: 2-D colour Doppler

On this apical four-chamber view, jets of both tricuspid and mitral regurgitation can be seen. Functional mitral regurgitation and tricuspid regurgitation are both common in dilated cardiomyopathy and are most commonly caused by dilatation of the valve rings. Colour Doppler can only be used in a semi-quantitative fashion to assess severity: in this case, the regurgitant jets are broad and reach the back of their respective atria, suggesting that regurgitation is severe.

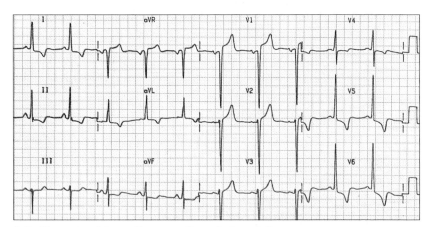

6.5 Hypertrophic cardiomyopathy: electrocardiogram

The chest radiograph is usually normal in hypertrophic cardiomyopathy. However, the ECG is nearly always abnormal with exaggerated voltage deflexions and ST segment and T wave changes reflecting LV hypertrophy. The changes are nonspecific, however, and may also occur in hypertrophic LV disease caused by hypertension or aortic stenosis. In this example, the sum of the S wave in V1 and R wave in V6 exceeds 35 mm (3.5 mV), fulfilling voltage criteria for LV hypertrophy. Note also the deep T wave inversion in the lateral leads, a common finding in hypertrophic heart disease.

6.6a–e Hypertrophic cardiomyopathy: echocardiogram

The echocardiogram is usually diagnostic of hypertrophic cardiomyopathy. LV hypertrophy (either regional or global) is invariable. Systolic anterior motion (SAM) of the mitral valve and mid-systolic closure of the aortic valve may also be present.

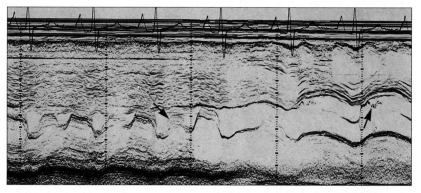

6.6a Hypertrophic cardiomyopathy: M-mode echocardiogram. Note the massive septal hypertrophy in excess of 3 cm with relatively normal posterior wall thickness. There is systolic anterior motion of the anterior mitral valve leaflet and midsystolic closure of the aortic valve (both arrowed), typical features that are commonly associated with LV outflow tract obstruction.

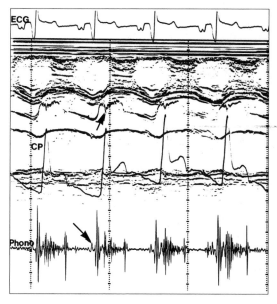

6.6b Hypertrophic cardiomyopathy: M-mode recording of aortic valve with simultaneous carotid pulse (CP) recording and phonocardiogram. Note the sharp upstroke to the CP with an abrupt decline in mid-systole associated with premature closure of the aortic valve (arrowed). The phonocardiogram shows the 4th heart sound (arrowed) and the systolic ejection murmur characteristic of the condition.

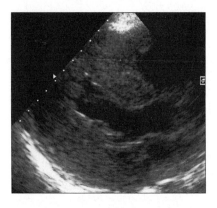

6.6c Hypertrophic cardiomyopathy: 2-D echocardiogram (long axis view). Note the gross LV hypertrophy, affecting both the interventricular septum and posterior wall.

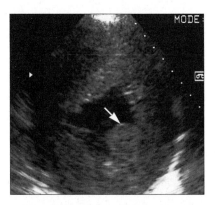

6.6d Hypertrophic cardiomyopathy: 2-D echocardiogram (short axis view). Note that the LV hypertrophy also involves the papillary muscles (arrowed).

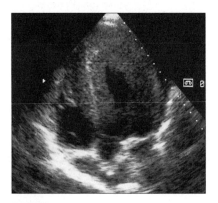

6.6e Hypertrophic cardiomyopathy: 2-D echocardiogram (four-chamber view). Again, severe LV hypertrophy is shown which in this example is global in distribution.

6.7 Hypertrophic cardiomyopathy: MRI

This coronal section shows severe hypertrophy of the LV wall with virtual obliteration of the cavity.

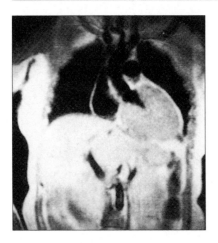

6.8a–d Hypertrophic cardiomyopathy: LV outflow tract obstruction

In many (not all) cases of hypertrophic cardiomyopathy, variable obstruction to the LV outflow tract occurs, caused by the bulky interventricular septum and the systolic anterior motion of the mitral valve leaflets. The obstruction is dynamic and can be provoked in certain patients by inotropic stimuli. This must be distinguished from the fixed outflow obstruction caused by aortic stenosis.

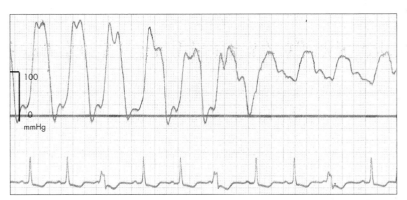

6.8a Hypertrophic cardiomyopathy: LV outflow tract obstruction. This is a pressure trace recorded as a catheter is pulled back from the LV cavity, through the LV outflow tract into the aortic root. Note the systolic pressure gradient of 50 mmHg in the LV outflow tract; there is no gradient across the aortic valve itself.

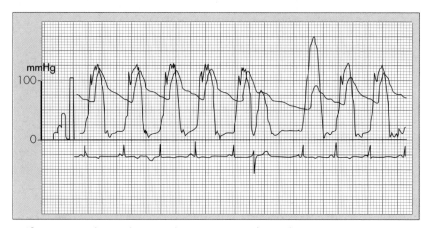

6.8b Hypertrophic cardiomyopathy: provocation of LV outflow gradient. Postextrasystolic 'potentiation' is a well-recognized inotropic stimulus which has been used therapeutically in heart failure. Here, simultaneous recordings of LV and aortic pressure signals show provocation of a gradient in the beat after a ventricular extrasystole. Contrast this with the finding in aortic stenosis where extrasystoles have no effect on the pressure gradient (5.6b).

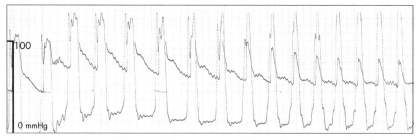

6.8c Hypertrophic cardiomyopathy: provocation of LV outflow tract gradient. The Valsalva manoeuvre provides another means of provoking LV outflow obstruction in hypertrophic cardiomyopathy. Here, simultaneous recording of the LV and aortic pressure signals before and during Valsalva shows provocation of a large pressure gradient. Contrast this with the effects of Valsalva in aortic stenosis in which the fixed pressure gradient across the valve is largely unaffected (see 6.8d).

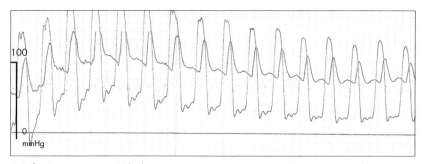

6.8d Aortic stenosis: Valsalva manoeuvre in aortic stenosis the pressure gradient is fixed. Here simultaneous recordings of the LV and aortic pressure signals before and during the Valsalva manoeuvre are shown with no increase in the pressure gradient.

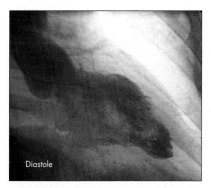
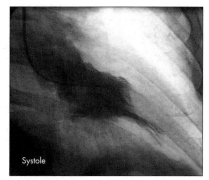

6.9 Hypertrophic cardiomyopathy: LV angiogram

Although relaxation is severely impaired in hypertrophic cardiomyopathy, the diastolic frame reveals relatively normal end diastolic volume. Systolic contraction, however, is hyperdynamic and in the systolic frame there is almost total obliteration of the LV cavity. This is particularly marked towards the apex in this example.

6.10a–e Restrictive cardiomyopathy

Restrictive cardiomyopathy is characterized physiologically by severely impaired ventricular relaxation in diastole. In this respect, it resembles constrictive pericarditis and differential diagnosis may be difficult.

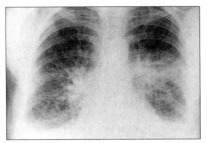

6.10a Restrictive cardiomyopathy: chest radiograph. The heart size is within normal limits but there is marked pulmonary congestion with a typical perihilar bat-wing distribution of pulmonary oedema.

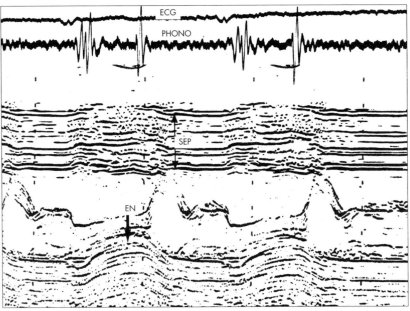

6.10b Restrictive cardiomyopathy: M-mode echocardiogram. The patient has cardiac amyloid. Note the marked hypertrophy of the septum (SEP) and posterior wall but low voltage complexes on the ECG. The endocardium (EN) and epicardium (EP) are indicated. Note the lack of systolic thickening and diastolic thinning of the posterior wall typical of cardiac amyloid.

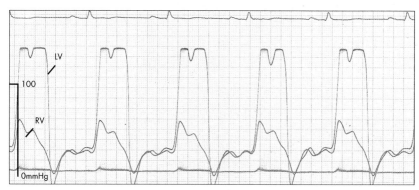

6.10c Restrictive cardiomyopathy: left and right ventricular pressure signals. Diastolic pressures rise and equalize (with loss of the normal differential) in order to maintain filling of the stiff ventricles. Note the typical dip and plateau (square root) appearance of the diastolic pressure signals.

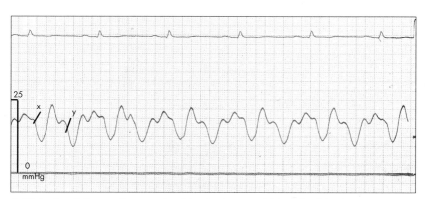

6.10d Restrictive cardiomyopathy: RA pressure signal. Note that RA pressure is elevated with prominence of both the 'x' and 'y' descents. Clinically, differentiation between these negative waves may be difficult but they give the jugular venous pulse an unusually dynamic appearance.

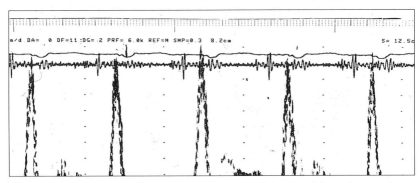

m/d DA= 0 DF=11 :DG= .2 PRF= 6.0k REF=H SMP=0.3 8.2cm   S= 12.5c

6.10e Restrictive cardiomyopathy: pulsed Doppler of transmitral flow. This reveals a very short LV filling time with rapid acceleration and deceleration. The short deceleration time of transmitral flow defines restrictive filling. Note that the forces required to accelerate blood flow across the mitral valve in these circumstances will be high and LA pressure will inevitably rise.

7.

Pericardial Disease

7.1a and b Pericarditis: ECG

In pericarditis, minor subepicardial injury produces ST elevation, affecting any or all of the ECG leads (except aVR) depending on the site of pericardial inflammation. The ST segments return to the baseline as the pericardial inflammation subsides.

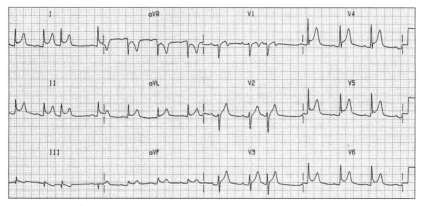

7.1a Pericarditis: ECG. This is a typical recording showing ST elevation with characteristic concave upwards morphology. Note the atrial ectopic beats, a common feature of Pericarditis.

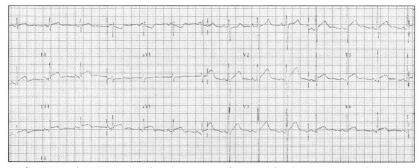

7.1b Pericarditis: ECG. Here the appearance is less typical with convex upwards ST elevation. Acute myocardial infarction has to be ruled out. The true diagnosis of pericarditis may only come to light over the course of time as the ST segment elevation fails to subside.

7.2 Pericardial cyst: chest radiograph

Pericardial cysts are not uncommon and are benign. No treatment is necessary.

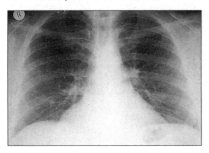

7.2a Pericardial cyst: chest radiograph. This is the typical appearance with a mass at the right cardiophrenic angle. It is commonly called a rain-water cyst because of the clear, watery appearance of the cystic fluid.

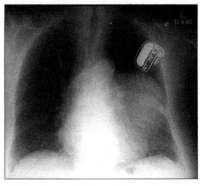

7.2b Pericardial cyst: chest radiograph. A large smooth mass at the left heart border is clearly visible. This is a giant pericardial cyst. In the absence of symptoms, no treatment is necessary.

7.3a and b Pericardial effusion with tamponade: ECG

The major causes of tamponade in this country are haemopericardium after heart surgery and pericardial effusion complicating neoplastic disease. Nevertheless, almost any other cause of pericardial haemorrhage or effusion may lead to tamponade, depending on the rate at which the fluid accumulates and, to a lesser extent, the volume of fluid.

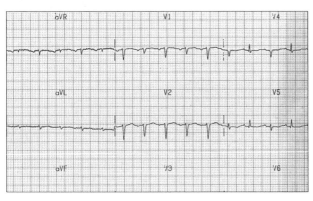

7.3a Pericardial effusion with tamponade: ECG. The voltage deflections are diminished. Note also 'electrical alternans' (beat–to–beat variation in R wave magnitude) reflecting an alternating electrical axis caused by movement of the heart within the fluid-filled pericardial sac.

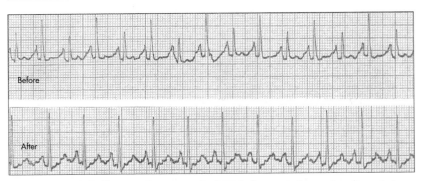

7.3b Pericardial effusion with tamponade: ECG before and after pericardiocentesis. Before pericardiocentesis, there is marked electrical alternans but afterwards, this disappears and the voltage deflections become more prominent.

7.4a–c Pericardial effusion with tamponade: chest radiograph

Pericardial effusion causes cardiac enlargement but diagnostic differentiation from other causes of cardiac enlargement cannot be made with confidence from the chest radiograph. Typically, however, pericardial effusion gives the cardiac silhouette a 'globular' appearance with an unusually crisp ('stencilled') edge because the parietal layer of the pericardial sac is immobilized by the effusion, eliminating movement artefact at the interface with the lung.

7.4a Pericardial effusion with tamponade: chest radiograph before and after pericardiocentesis.

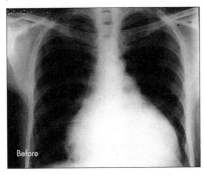

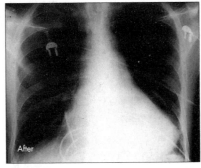

7.4a(i) Before pericardiocentesis, the cardiac silhouette is enlarged and globular.

7.4a(ii) A pig-tail catheter was inserted by the subxiphistern route to drain the effusion, after which the heart size was reduced. The tip of the catheter is seen lying in the pericardial sac behind the left heart border.

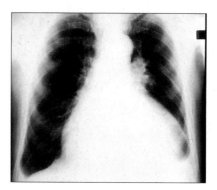

7.4b   Pericardial effusion with tamponade: chest radiograph. There is a left hilar mass caused by carcinoma. Pericardial infiltration has produced effusion and tamponade shown by the severe cardiac enlargement. Malignant disease is now one of the most common causes of tamponade in the UK.

7.4c(i) and (ii)   Pericardial effusion with tamponade: chest radiograph.

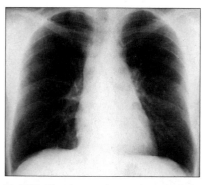

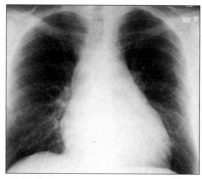

7.4c(i)   The chest radiograph on the left reveals bilateral hilar lymph node enlargement but a normal cardiac size. This was caused by tuberculosis and over the following 2 weeks a tuberculous pericardial effusion developed.

7.4c(ii)   The panel on the right reveals a markedly enlarged cardiac shadow with a globular shape, indicating pericardial effusion.

7.5a–e   Pericardial effusion with tamponade: echocardiogram
Echocardiography is the most sensitive technique available for the diagnosis of pericardial effusion. The effusion appears as an echo-free space distributed around the ventricles but usually avoiding the potential space behind the left atrium.

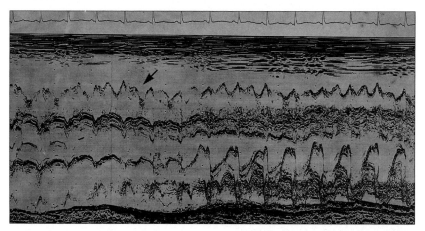

7.5a Pericardial effusion with tamponade: M-mode echocardiogram. Note the echo-free space in front of and behind the heart, caused by pericardial effusion. There is diastolic inward motion of the right ventricular free wall (arrowed).

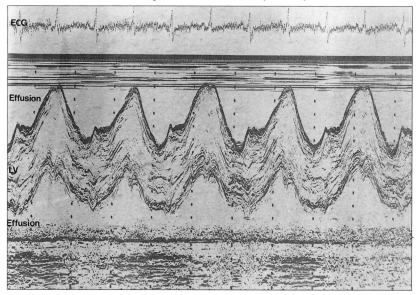

7.5b Pericardial effusion with tamponade: M-mode echocardiogram. Severe tamponade caused by large anterior and posterior pericardial effusions has all but obliterated the right ventricular cavity. The heart is swinging around within the effusion and the simultaneous ECG shows electrical alternans.

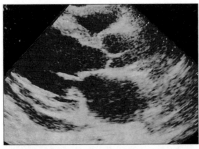

7.5c Pericardial effusion with tamponade: 2-D echocardiogram (parasternal long axis view). Note the echo-free space around the heart but not behind the left atrium. The effusion was small but in this case developed rapidly and was sufficient to cause tamponade within the noncompliant pericardial sac.

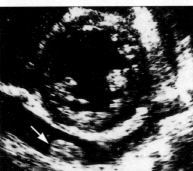

7.5d Pericardial effusion with tamponade: 2-D echocardiogram (parasternal short axis view). There is an effusion surrounding the heart. The patient had severe chicken pox, and the mass in the pericardial space posteriorly (arrowed) could represent a pox lesion.

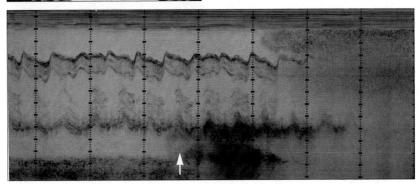

7.5e Pericardial effusion with tamponade: M-mode echocardiogram during pericardiocentesis. A large effusion is visible as an echo-free space around the heart. In order to confirm that the drainage catheter was correctly sited before aspirating the effusion, a small amount of agitated saline was injected into the pericardial space at the time indicated by the arrow. The catheter tip was sitting posteriorly; dense echoes are seen first behind the heart but soon come to surround it, effectively obliterating the echocardiographic image and confirming that the drainage catheter was correctly sited within the pericardial space.

7.6a–d Pericardial tamponade: haemodynamics

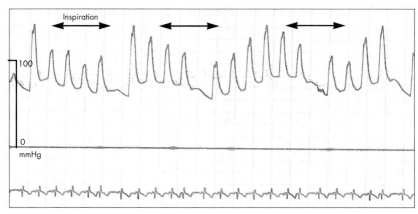

7.6a Pericardial tamponade: pulsus paradoxus (radial artery pressure signal). Note the exaggerated (>10 mmHg) decline in arterial pressure during inspiration. Pulsus paradoxus is nearly always present in tamponade but may occur in constrictive pericarditis, severe obstructive airways disease and tension pneumothorax.

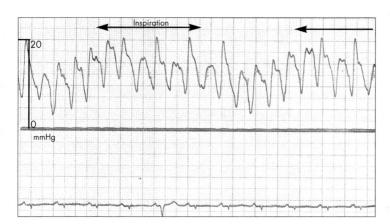

7.6b Pericardial tamponade: jugular venous pressure. The venous pressure is raised and there are prominent 'x' and 'y' descents, giving the waveform of the JVP an unusually dynamic appearance. Note the inspiratory rise in atrial pressure (Kussmaul's sign), reflecting the inability of the tamponaded right heart to accommodate the inspiratory increase in venous return.

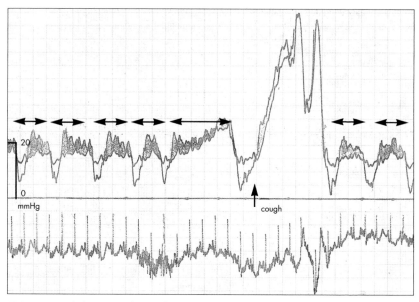

7.6c Pericardial tamponade: simultaneous right atrial and pulmonary capillary wedge pressure signals. In tamponade, intrapericardial pressure rises and restricts cardiac filling. The thin–walled RV is worst affected. A compensatory rise in RV filling pressure occurs which comes to equal LV filling pressure. Thereafter, filling pressures of both ventricles rise together as tamponade increases. This is reflected in these simultaneous recordings of the right atrial and pulmonary capillary wedge pressures (the RV and LV filling pressures, respectively) which are effectively superimposed. Note that during inspiration (arrows) RA pressure rises (Kussmaul's sign) but pulmonary capillary wedge pressure is unaffected. When the patient coughs (arrowed) the transient rise in intrathoracic pressure produces a corresponding rise in both pressure signals, which remain superimposed.

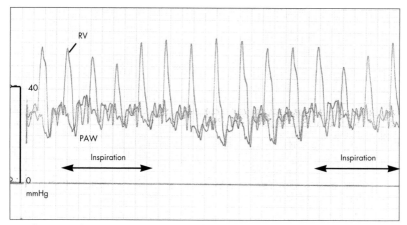

7.6d Pericardial tamponade: simultaneous recordings of the right ventricular and pulmonary capillary wedge pressures. Note the equalization and elevation of RV diastolic and PA wedge pressures (the RV and LV filling pressures, respectively) and also that during inspiration, RV filling pressure increases (Kussmaul's sign) and peak systolic pressure declines (pulsus paradoxus).

7.7a–c Pericardial constriction: chest radiograph

The chest radiograph is often normal in pericardial constriction. Indeed, the combination of a normal chest radiograph and signs of severe right-sided failure is suggestive of the diagnosis. So is the presence of pericardial calcification (best seen on the lateral projection), although this is seen in <50% of patients.

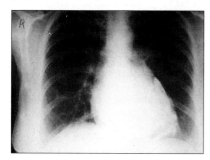

7.7a Pericardial constriction: postero-anterior chest radiograph. Pericardial calcification is seen clearly but a lateral projection is usually more useful.

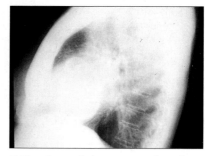

7.7b Pericardial constriction: lateral chest radiograph. Pericardial calcification is seen around the front and the back of the heart.

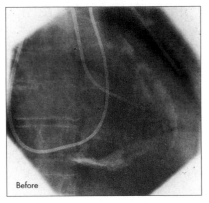 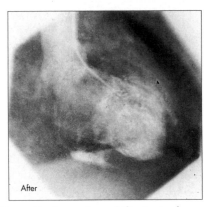

Before   After

7.7c Pericardial constriction: fluoroscopy. Radiographically, cardiac calcification is often best seen by fluoroscopy in the catheter laboratory. This LV angiogram (before and after contrast injection) clearly shows a calcified.

7.8a–d Pericardial constriction: CT and MRI scans

CT scanning is probably the best imaging technique for measuring pericardial thickness and is commonly used for diagnosis of constriction. MRI can provide similar information.

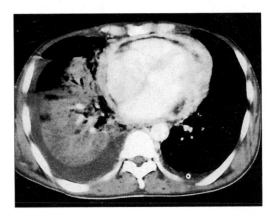

7.8a Noncalcific pericardial constriction: CT scan. Consolidation in the right lung and severe pericardial thickening are present. The patient had pulmonary tuberculosis with pericardial involvement and presented with fever and signs of constriction. Antituberculous therapy caused regression of all symptoms and signs, although the patient is at major risk of developing constriction later as the pericardium becomes fibrotic and calcified.

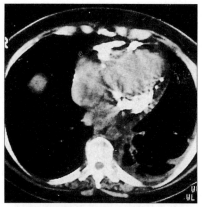

7.8b Calcific pericardial constriction: CT scan. There is dense calcification of the pericardium, which is white with an appearance similar to bone. This patient had had tuberculosis several years previously.

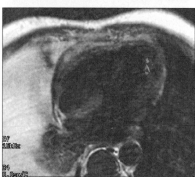

7.8c Pericardial constriction: MRI scan (transverse section). Severe noncalcific pericardial thickening is evident, particularly over the lateral and apical walls of the heart.

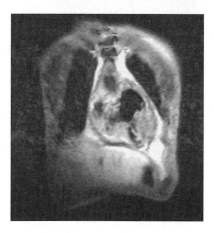

7.8d Pericardial constriction: MRI scan (coronal section). Severe calcific pericardial thickening is evident, surrounding the heart.

7.9 Pericardial constriction: haemodynamics

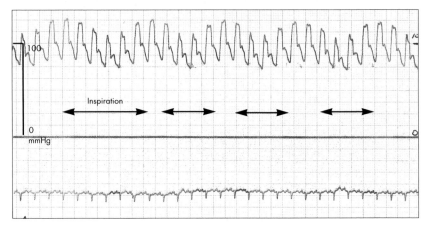

7.9a Pericardial constriction: aortic pressure signal. Paradox is rarely as marked in constriction as it is in tamponade. In this example, there is only mild to moderate respiratory variation in aortic pressure, never exceeding 15mmHg.

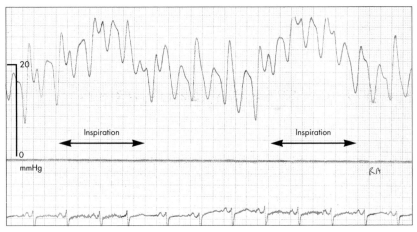

7.9b Pericardial constriction: RA pressure signal. The pressure is elevated and prominence of the 'x' and 'y' descents is clearly visible. There is phasic variation in pressure, which rises during inspiration (Kussmaul's sign), reflecting the inability of the constricted right heart to accommodate the inspiratory increase in venous return. Kussmaul's sign is almost invariable in pericardial constriction.

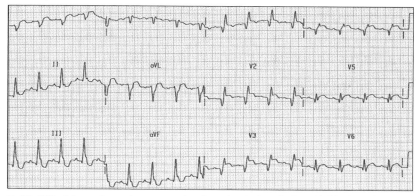

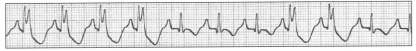

9.7c Intermittent bundle branch block. It is important to recognize that bundle branch block may be intermittent, as shown in this example.

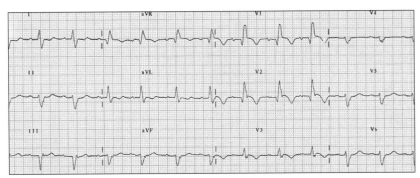

9.7d Bifascicular block (RBBB and left axis deviation). Isolated block in either the anterior or posterior division of the left bundle is called hemiblock and produces left or right axis deviation, respectively. When hemiblock is associated with RBBB, bifascicular block results when AV conduction is dependent on the remaining division of the left bundle. The danger of complete AV block developing is appreciable particularly in AMI when prophylactic pacemaker therapy is indicated. This example, shows RBBB and left axis deviation with a prolonged PA interval.

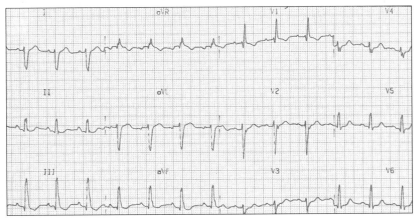

9.7e Bifascicular block (RBBB and right axis deviation). Here, right bundle branch block is associated with right axis deviation.

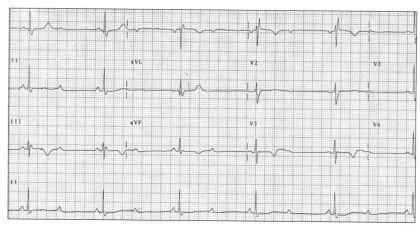

9.7f Mobitz type 2 AV block. This always indicates advanced conduction tissue disease affecting the bundle branches. Note that the PR interval of conducted beats is normal but the QRS complex shows right bundle branch block. Intermittent block in the left bundle results in failure of conduction of alternate P waves. Permanent pacing is mandatory because if bilateral bundle branch block is prolonged, reliable escape rhythms cannot be depended on.

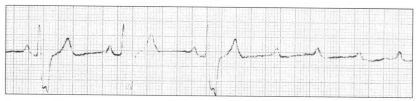

9.7g Mobitz type 2 AV block. The first three QRS complexes show a bundle branch block pattern with a normal PR interval. However, the T waves are distorted by nonconducted P waves, reflecting intermittent block in the other bundle branch. At the end of the strip, bilateral bundle branch block persists resulting in a long run of asystole. This emphasizes the importance of permanent pacing in Mobitz type 2 block.

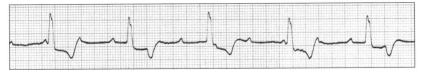

9.7h   Complete heart block: bundle branch level. The atrial and ventricular rhythms are dissociated because none of the atrial impulses is conducted. The ECG shows regular P waves and regular but slower QRS complexes. The escape rhythm is ventricular in origin therefore the QRS complexes are broad and the rate is slow. The risk of prolonged asystole is significant and permanent pacing is mandatory.

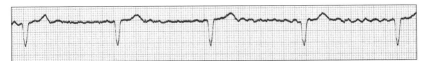

9.7i   Complete heart block: bundle branch level. In this example, the atrium is fibrillating and AV dissociation is, therefore, less apparent than in previous examples. However, the QRS complexes are slow, regular and broad, indicating that this is a ventricular escape rhythm in a patient with bilateral bundle branch block. Again, permanent pacing is mandatory.

Methods of pacing: five-letter code				
Chamber paced	**Chamber sensed**	**Response to sensing**	**Programming and rate responsiveness**	**Anti-tachycardia capability**
O = None	O = None	O = None	O = None	O = None
A = Atrium	A = Atrium	T = Triggered	P = Simple	P = Pacing
V = Ventricle	V = Ventricle	I = Inhibited	M = Multiprogrammable	S = Shock
D = Dual (A+V)	D = Dual (A+V)	D = Dual (T+I)	C = Communicating	P = Dual (P+S)
			R = Rate responsive	

9.8   Cardiac pacing: five-letter code

An international five-letter code describes the various methods of pacing. For practical purposes, however, only the first three letters are usually used, describing the chamber paced, the chamber sensed and the mode of response to sensing. The fourth letter, R, is applied when the unit is rate responsive, permitting a physiological increase in heart rate with exercise. The fifth letter is rarely used. The most widely used pacing methods are AAI, VVI, DDD and DDI. Any of these may be rate responsive; if so R maybe added.

Indications for pacing and preferred mode		
Disorder	**Indication for pacing**	**Preferred pacing mode**
Sin-oatrial disease	Symptomatic bradycardias (possibly a consequence of necessary anti-arrhythmic drug therapy)	AAI(R)* if no evidence of AV node or bundle branch disease
		DDD(R)* if concomitant AV node disease
		VVIR for patients with AF or frequent paroxysmal arrhythmias
Atrioventricular block (junctional level)	Symptomatic complete or 2° block	DDD(R)*
		VVIR for patients with AF or frequent paroxysmal arrhythmias
Intraventricular AV block (bundle branch level)	Symptomatic complete or 2° block	DDD(R)*
	Asymptomatic complete or Mobitz type 2 block	VVIR for patients with AF or frequent paroxysmal arrhythmias
	Symptomatic chronic bifascicular block (caused by intermittent complete block)	
	Acute bifascicular block complicating myocardial infarction	

* Rate responsive units required for patients with chronotropic incompetence

9.9 Cardiac pacing

The table shows indications for pacing and the preferred pacing mode for patients with sino–atrial disease, atrioventricular block at junctional level and atrioventricular block at bundle branch level.

9.10a and b Cardiac pacing: chest radiograph

A chest radiograph must always be obtained after implantation of a permanent pacemaker system, to confirm that the wire is properly positioned and there is no pneumothorax.

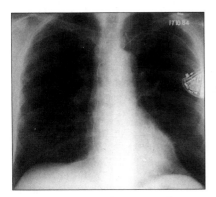

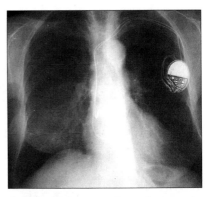

9.10a VVI pacemaker system. The power source (or generator) is positioned subcutaneously in the left pectoral position below the left clavicle and attached to a wire with a terminal electrode positioned in the apex of the right ventricle.

9.10b DDD pacing. Again the generator is in the left pectoral position, but here is attached to two wires positioned respectively in the right atrium and right ventricle.

9.11a–c Cardiac pacing: ECG

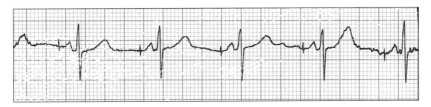

9.11a AAI pacing. The pacing electrode is positioned in the right atrial appendage. The atrium is sensed and spontaneous contractions inhibit the pacemaker. Thus, pacing only occurs during atrial standstill to prevent prolonged asystolic pauses. Note the pacing artefact that precedes each P wave. Clearly, AAI pacing cannot be used in patients with AV block. However, it is the method of choice in patients with isolated sino–atrial disease in whom AV conduction is normal.

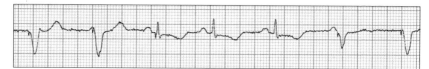

9.11b VVI pacing. This is still the most commonly used method of pacing even though it is no longer the method of choice in the majority of patients. The pacing electrode is positioned in the right ventricle. Spontaneous ventricular beats are sensed and inhibit the pulse generator. Thus, the pacemaker is only activated when the spontaneous ventricular rate falls below the preselected pacing rate. Here, the first two complexes are paced but there follow three sinus beats that inhibit the pacemaker. Thereafter, the sinus rate slows and ventricular pacing is resumed.

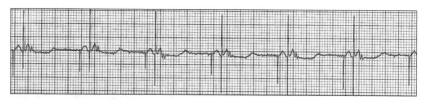

9.11c DDD pacing. This is a dual-chamber pacing method with pacing electrodes positioned in the right atrium and right ventricle. DDD pacing re-establishes a normal AV relationship by delivering impulses with physiological delay first to the right atrium and then to the ventricle. Alternatively, if normal atrial activity is intact it may be sensed by the atrial lead and trigger ventricular stimulation, again with appropriate delay. Clearly, DDD pacing cannot be used in patients with atrial fibrillation. In this example, sequential atrial and ventricular DDD pacing is illustrated.

10.

Disease of Thoracic Aorta

10.1 Degenerative aortic disease of elderly individuals

The aorta tends to lengthen with age and show variable dilatation. This unfolding process is benign and does not affect aortic function. Atheroma preferentially affects the proximal aorta but unlike the smaller coronary and cerebral vessels rarely causes significant obstruction.

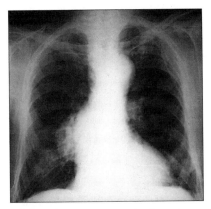

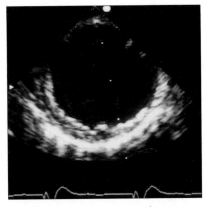

10.1a Degenerative aortic disease: chest radiograph showing unfolded aorta. Note that elongation of the thoracic aorta has caused it to to take a serpentine course through the superior mediastinum and behind the heart.

10.1b Degenerative aortic disease: transoesophageal echocardiogram (horizontal plane) showing atheroma. Note the thickening and irregularity of the aortic intima and media and the extensive atheromatous plaque extending from 4–9 o'clock in the descending aorta.

10.2a–g Aortic aneurysm

Aortic aneurysms occur most commonly in the abdominal aorta, where they are usually the result of atherosclerosis. Aneurysms of the descending thoracic aorta are also atherosclerotic in most cases but in the ascending aorta, Marfan's syndrome and other causes of cystic medial necrosis have replaced syphilis as the most common cause. Thoracic aortic aneurysms involving the aortic root often cause aortic regurgitation. Rupture is unusual but may occur in large (or rapidly enlarging) aneurysms. Thus, regular monitoring (usually by echocardiography) is essential, particularly in young patients with Marfan's syndrome.

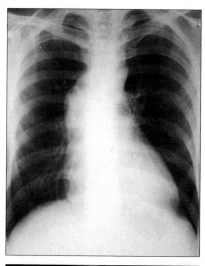

10.2a Aortic aneurysm: chest radiograph. Note the dilatation of the ascending aorta in this patient with Marfan's syndrome.

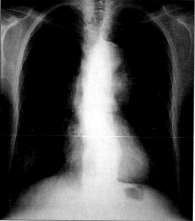

10.2b Aortic aneurysm: chest radiograph (PA projection). Note the large calcified aneurysm involving the aortic arch.

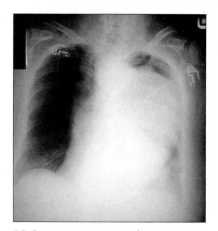

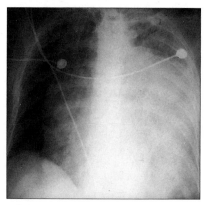

10.2c Aortic aneurysm: chest radiograph (PA projection). Note the hugely dilated aortic arch and descending aorta occupying almost the entire left hemithorax.

10.2d Aortic aneurysm: chest radiograph (portable film, AP projection). Ruptured thoracic aortic aneurysm with extravasation of blood into the mediastinum and pleural spaces. The patient died shortly after this radiograph was taken.

10.2e(i) and (ii) Aortic aneurysm: 2-D echocardiogram. The patient had Marfan's syndrome.

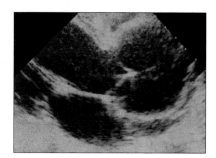

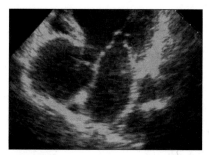

10.2e(i) The parasternal long axis view reveals marked dilatation of the aortic root immediately above the valve.

10.2e(ii) The apical view reveals the full extent of the aneurysm involving the sinuses of Valsalva and proximal ascending aorta.

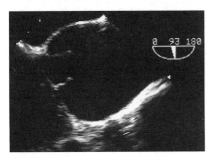

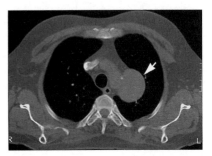

10.2f Aortic aneurysm: transoesophageal echocardiogram (longitudinal plane). Another patient with Marfan's syndrome. The flask-like dilatation of the aortic root is clearly seen.

10.2g Aortic aneurysm: CT scan. This aneurysm was a deceleration injury caused by a road traffic accident. The scan shows a large aneurysm of the aortic arch (arrowed) arising just after the left subclavian branch. This is the typical location for deceleration aortic aneurysms.

10.3a–n Aortic dissection

As with aortic aneurysm, aortic dissection is caused by disease of the aortic media, often atherosclerosis or cystic medial necrosis as seen in Marfan's syndrome. Patients are often hypertensive, particularly when the dissection arises in the aortic arch. More proximal dissections involving the aortic root commonly cause aortic regurgitation. Diagnosis of dissection requires an imaging modality that shows the intimal flap separating true and false aortic lumens. Transoesophageal echocardiography and CT scanning have emerged as the imaging modalities of choice for diagnosis.

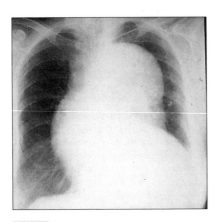

10.3a (i) Aortic dissection: chest radiograph. Note the widened mediastium with left pleural effusion. These are 'classical' radiographic findings in the dissection of the thoracic aorta.

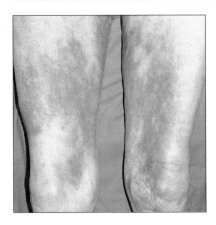

10.3a (ii) Aortic dissection. In this patient, blood flow to the lower limbs was compromised: dissection of the descending aorta down into the iliac vessels caused severe ischaemia of both legs.

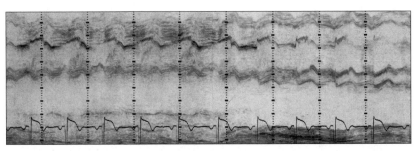

10.3b Aortic dissection: M-mode echocardiogram. M-mode echocardiography is not often helpful in dissection but in this example the aortic root is dilated and the intimal flap is clearly visible within the lumen.

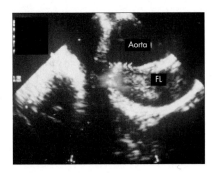

10.3c Aortic dissection: transoesophageal echocardiogram. This is the ultrasound imaging modality of choice. Here the flap is visible as an echo-dense line across the centre of the aortic lumen, with false lumen (FL) below. There is spontaneous contrast suggestive of sluggish flow in the false lumen and a colour Doppler jet of flow into the false lumen through the intimal tear can be clearly seen.

10.3d(i) and (ii)   Aortic dissection: transoesophageal echocardiogram.

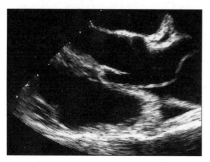

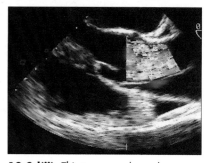

10.3d(i) This longitudinal axis transoesophageal echocardiogram reveals the dilated aortic root and an S-shaped flap traversing the lumen.

10.3d(ii) This transoesophageal echocardiogram of the same patient with colour Doppler superimposed to show flow in the true lumen.

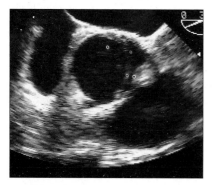

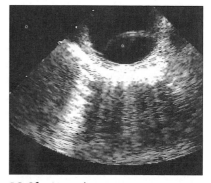

10.3e Aortic dissection: transoesophageal echocardiogram. Note the dilated aortic root with a vertical line indicative of a flap. The flap divides the aortic lumen into a larger false lumen on the left and a smaller true lumen on the right. The right coronary artery is seen arising from the false lumen, and the left main coronary artery from the true lumen.

10.3f Aortic dissection: transoesophageal echocardiogram of the descending aorta. The intimal flap is clearly shown, indicating dissection down into the descending aorta.

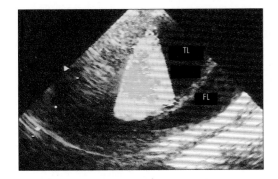

10.3g Aortic dissection: transoesophageal echocardiogram. The aortic arch is shown with an intimal flap dividing the true lumen (TL) from the false (FL) lumen. Colour flow Doppler defines the true lumen.

10.3h Aortic dissection: CT scan.

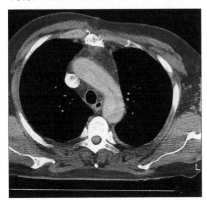

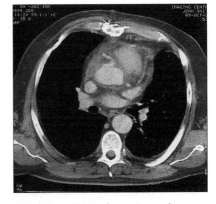

10.3h(i) CT scan: aortic arch. An intimal flap is seen as a radiolucent line within the aortic lumen.

10.3h(ii) CT scan: heart. External rupture into the pericardial space has produced a large haematoma surrounding the heart. This is often fatal and prompt surgery is usually necessary.

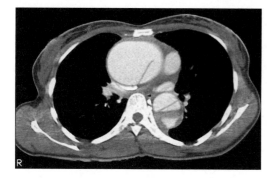

10.3i Aortic dissection: CT scan (Marfan's syndrome). The ascending aorta is severely dilated and the intimal flap is clearly visible. This flap extends around the arch (not shown) and further into the descending aorta where, again, it is clearly visible.

10.3j (i) and (ii)   Aortic dissection: MRI scan.

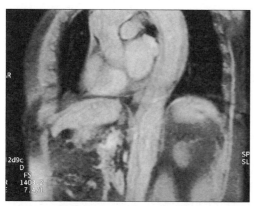

10.3j (i) Coronal section showing an extensive aortic dissection extending from the aortic root through the arch and into the descending aorta. The lower panel reveals a transverse view through the heart and descending aorta.

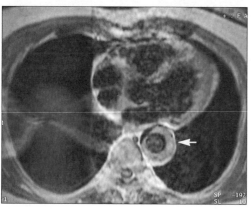

10.3j (ii) Transverse section through the heart and descending aorta. Note the circumferencal false lumen filled with clot in the descending aorta (arrowed).

10.3k(i) and (ii)   Aortic dissection: MRI scan (transverse plane).

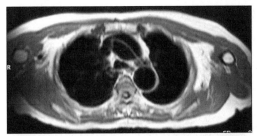

10.3k(i) Ascending thoracic aorta. The intimal flap is clearly visible.

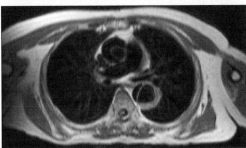

10.3k(ii) Descending thoracic aorta. The dissection has extended into the descending aorta where the intimal flap is clearly visible.

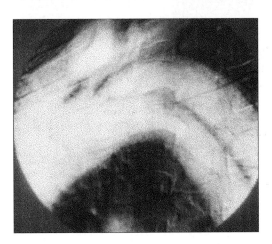

10.3l Aortic dissection: digital subtraction angiogram. Abrupt widening of the aorta occurs after the left subclavian branch. The intimal flap is clearly visible.

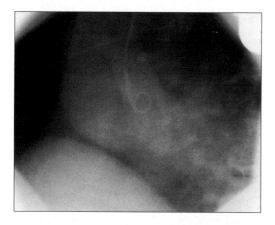

10.3m Aortic dissection: aortogram. There is a pigtail catheter in a dilated aortic root and the line of an aortic dissection can be seen within the aortic lumen. Aortography is now rarely performed to make a diagnosis of dissection, which is usually confirmed with either CT scan, transoesophageal echocardiography or MRI scanning.

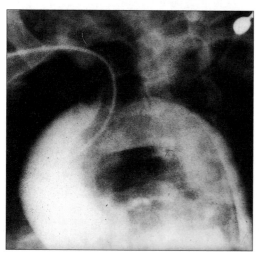

10.3n Aortic dissection: aortogram. The aortic root is dilated with an intimal flap within the sinuses of Valsalva (note the aortic regurgitation), extending down the thoracic aorta.

10.4a–d Sinus of Valsalva aneurysm

Sinus of Valsalva aneurysm may be mycotic, occurring as a complication of infective endocarditis. More commonly, it is congenital usually affecting the right coronary sinus. Progressive aneurysmal bulging of the affected sinus may lead to rupture into a right-sided cardiac chamber (usually right ventricle), resulting in an arteriovenous shunt.

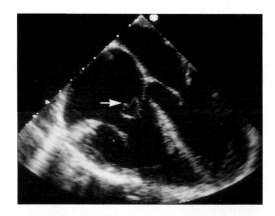

10.4a Sinus of Valsalva aneurysm: transoesophageal echocardiogram showing rupture into right atrium. This horizontal plane image (four-chamber view) shows a dilated right atrium and right ventricle. Within the right atrium there is a circular ring shadow (arrowed) representing the end of the sinus of Valsalva aneurysm in the fashion of a 'wind-sock'.

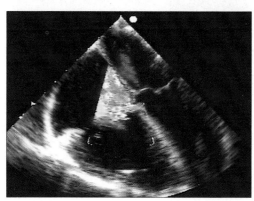

10.4b Sinus of Valsalva aneurysm: transoesophageal echocardiogram. This colour flow Doppler study reveals turbulent flow from the ruptured sinus of Valsalva aneurysm into the right atrium.

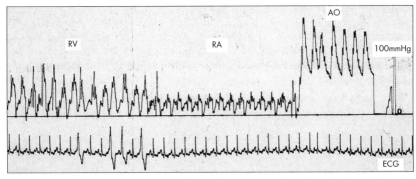

10.4c Sinus of Valsalva aneurysm: cardiac catheterization. The catheter has been directed into the right ventricle from the aorta through a ruptured aneurysm. The pressure signals have been recorded during pullback from the right ventricle into the right atrium and then into the aorta through the ruptured aneurysm.

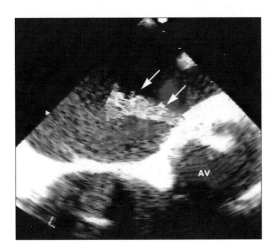

10.4d Sinus of Valsalva aneurysm caused by infective endocarditis: transoesophageal echocardiogram. A fistula had developed as a complication of infective endocarditis affecting, a xenograft valve placed in the aortic position. A colour flow Doppler jet (arrowed) of turbulent flow from the aortic root into the left atrium is shown.

11.

Adult Congenital Disease

11.1a–e Coarctation of the aorta

Coarctation is a localized fibrotic narrowing of the aorta, nearly always just beyond the origin of the left subclavian branch. It is more common in men and may be associated with bicuspid aortic valve, Berry aneurysm or gonadal dysgenesis (Turner's syndrome). It does not cause significant obstruction until the ductus arteriosus constricts after birth when acute LVF may occur. More commonly, heart failure is avoided by compensatory LV hypertrophy, providing time for development of an extensive collateral supply around the coarctation. Hypertension in the upper part of the body is almost invariable and predisposes to LVF and aortic dissection. Survival beyond the age of 40 years rarely occurs unless coarctation is surgically corrected.

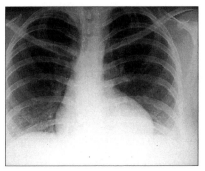

11.1a Coarctation of the aorta: chest radiograph. Note the notching of the inferior rib margins, the result of erosion by dilated intercostal collaterals.

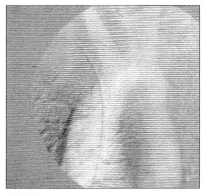

11.1b Coarctation of the aorta: digital subtraction arch aortogram. The coarctation is clearly visible in the descending thoracic aorta, just distal to the left subclavian branch.

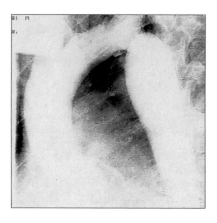

11.1c Coarctation of the aorta: arch aortogram. The coarctation is clearly visible just distal to the left subclavian branch.

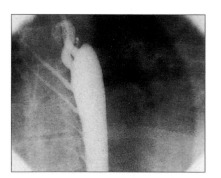

11.1d Coarctation of the aorta: aortogram. Contrast has been injected through a catheter advanced backwards from the leg into the thoracic aorta. In this patient, the thoracic aorta was completely occluded by the coarctation. Note the large collaterals feeding into the distal aorta. These are responsible for the rib notching commonly seen on the chest radiograph.

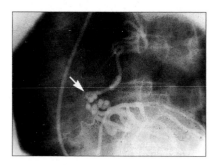

11.1e Coarctation of the aorta: left coronary arteriogram. In this unusual case, coronary arteriography revealed a leash of collaterals (arrowed) arising from the proximal left coronary system.

11.2a and b Pulmonary stenosis

Pulmonary stenosis is one of the most common congenital anomalies. Mild to moderate stenosis (peak systolic pressure gradient < 75 mmHg) is only rarely symptomatic. More severe cases may present in infancy with cyanosis and heart failure but, more commonly, present in later life with exertional dyspnoea progressing to RV failure. Treatment is by balloon dilatation of the pulmonary valve.

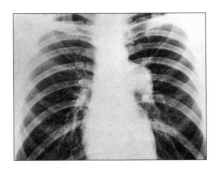

11.2a   Pulmonary stenosis: chest radiograph. Note the post–stenotic dilatation of the pulmonary artery.

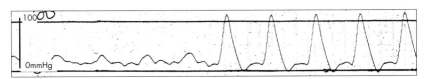

11.2b   Pulmonary stenosis: cardiac catherization. The cardiac catheter has been pulled back from the pulmonary artery across the pulmonary valve into the right ventricle. There is a peak gradient of about 80 mmHg, indicating moderately severe pulmonary stenosis.

11.3a–h   Atrial septal defect

Communications between the atria may be caused by sinus venosus defects high in the septum or 'primum' defects lower in the septum, which are often associated with anomalous pulmonary venous drainage and mitral valve abnormalities, respectively. The most common atrial septal defect (ASD), however, is the 'secundum' defect of the oval fossa. Blood shunts preferentially from left to right through the defect into the low resistance pulmonary circulation. Increased pulmonary flow predisposes to obliterative pulmonary vascular disease. In the majority of patients, however, an ASD remains asymptomatic at least until middle age, when presentation is usually with atrial fibrillation and symptoms of mild heart failure. For most patients, treatment is unnecessary but if the shunt is very large and symptoms severe, closure may be helpful.

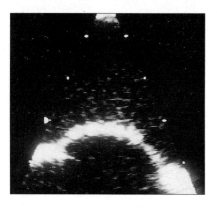

11.3a Atrial septum: transoesophageal echocardiogram of normal oval fossa. The ovale fossa sits centrally in the atrial septum and has a typical bowed appearance as shown here.

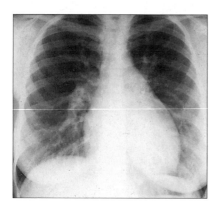

11.3b Atrial septal defect: patent foramen ovale. In a number of individuals the foramen ovale does not close completely. In this bubble-contrast study, the patent foramen is visible with contrast passing across it. Patency of the foramen ovale is rarely of any consequence unless paradoxical embolism occurs, resulting in stroke.

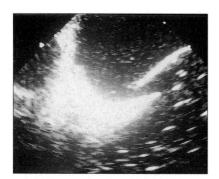

11.3c Atrial septal defect: chest radiograph. Note the prominent proximal pulmonary arteries and the pulmonary plethora reflecting increased pulmonary flow.

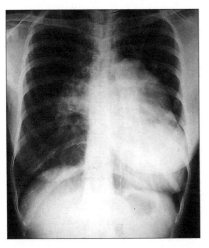

11.3d Atrial septal defect: chest radiograph. Here, the ASD has produced severe pulmonary hypertension as a result of obliterative pulmonary vascular disease. There is gross dilatation of the pulmonary arteries but because pulmonary flow is reduced there is no pulmonary plethora.

11.3e (i) and (ii) Atrial septal defect: 2-D echocardiogram (subcostal view).

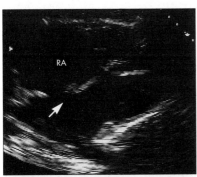

11.3e(i) In the subcostal view, good images of the interatrial septum can usually be obtained without resorting to transoesophageal echocardiography. Note the ASD (arrowed) and the dilatation of the right atrium (RA).

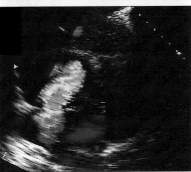

11.3e(ii) The colour flow Doppler confirms flow across the atrial septal defect.

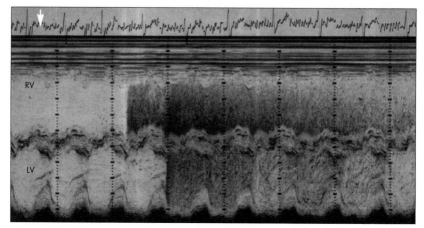

11.3f Atrial septal defect: M-mode echocardiogram with bubble contrast. Hand-agitated saline solution has been injected into a peripheral vein at the time indicated by the arrow. Bubble contrast appears first in the right side of the heart. Opacification of the left side of the heart is also seen, caused by passage of bubbles through an ASD. Note the relative dilatation of the right ventricle compared with the left ventricle.

11.3g Atrial septal defect: 2-D echocardiogram with bubble contrast.

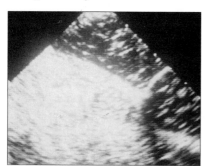

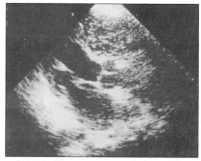

11.3g(i) ASD present. In this transoesophageal echocardiogram, bubble contrast is visible on both sides of the atrial septum confirming the presence of a defect.

11.3g (ii) ASD absent. In this transthoracic study (long axis view), bubble contrast is seen clearly in the right side of the heart but not on the left side, ruling out ASD.

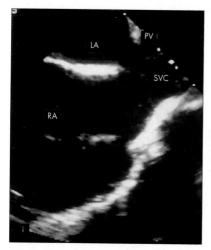 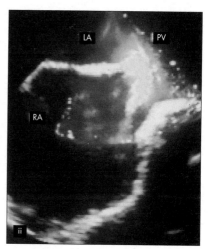

11.3h(i) and (ii)   Atrial septal defect: transoesophgeal echocardiogram(a) with colour Doppler(b). This is a sinus venosus defect (arrowed) high in the atrial septum at the junction with the superior vena cava (SVC). The colour Doppler study confirms free flow across the defect.

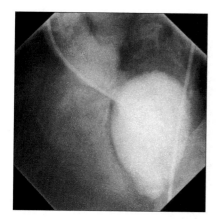

11.4   Ventricular septal defect

Ventricular septal defect (VSD) is a common congenital anomaly. Defects usually occur high in the septum in its perimembranous portion. Appoximately 40% close spontaneously in early childhood. Small defects that persist rarely cause symptoms, although they do predispose to endocarditis. Larger defects should be closed because they may be complicated by obliterative pulmonary vascular disease or LV failure. This illustration shows an LV angiogram in an adult. Note the VSD high in the interventricular septum with contrast crossing into the right ventricle.

11.5a(i) and (ii) **Patent ductus arteriosus**

Patency of the ductus arteriosus after birth produces a left to right shunt. Large shunts should be closed because they may cause heart failure in infancy or lead to obliterative pulmonary vascular disease.

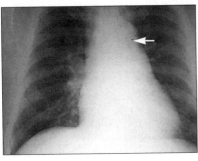

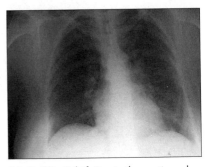

11.5a(i) Patent ductus arteriosus: chest radiograph. The chest radiograph is rarely of diagnostic value unless the duct is calcified as shown here (arrowed). Note that the calcified ductus is remote from the wall of the aorta.

11.5a(ii) Calcifation in the aortic arch. In contrast with the previous x–ray, the calcification in this example clearly lies within the wall of the aorta.

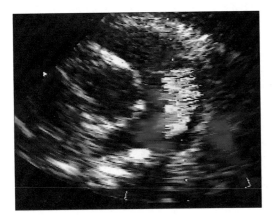

11.5b Patent ductus arteriosus: transoesophageal echocardiogram with colour Doppler. The pulmonary artery is shown curving around the aorta. Note that the pulmonary artery is dilated. The Doppler study shows turbulent flow in relation to patent ductus.

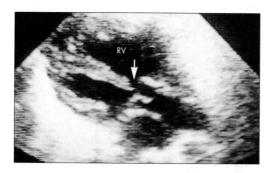

11.6 Tetralogy of Fallot

The tetralogy consists of subvalvar pulmonary outflow obstruction, ventricular septal defect, over-riding of the aorta and RV hypertrophy. Depending largely on the severity of RV outflow obstruction, blood shunts from right to left across the VSD. In severe obstruction, the shunt is large and cyanosis severe but in mild obstruction, pulmonary flow may be close to normal and shunting negligible (acyanotic Fallot's). Nevertheless, the outflow obstruction is often progressive and cyanosis usually develops during early childhood. Death in infancy may occur but less severely affected patients survive to adulthood, although survival beyond middle age is rare without surgical correction. This 2-D echocardiogram shows the VSD (arrowed) with the dilated aorta over-riding the defect. The right ventricle (RV) is significantly dilated.

11.7a and b Congential aortic stenosis

Congenital aortic stenosis is caused by commisural fusion which results in a bicuspid valve. It may present in infancy with severe aortic stenosis but, more commonly, stenosis remains trivial until adulthood when the valve calcifies. Treatment is the same as for other causes of aortic stenosis.

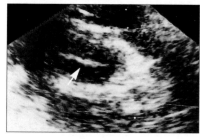

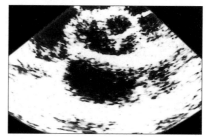

11.7a(i) Congenital aortic stenosis: 2-D echocardiogram. The bicuspid valve produces a single closure line (arrowed) across the aorta. .

11.7a(ii) Normal aortic valve. Note the three cusps producing a 'mercedes–Benz' configuration.

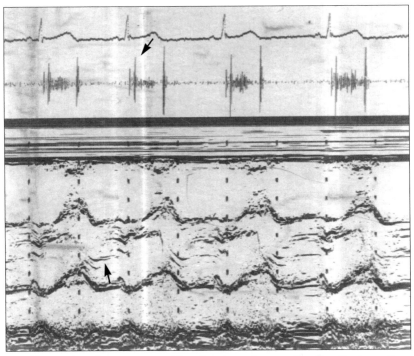

11.7b Congenital aortic stenosis: M-mode echocardiogram. The diastolic closure line of the aortic valve (arrowed) lies eccentrically within the aortic root, suggesting a bicuspid valve. The valve is normal in other respects. The ejection click (arrowed) and murmur typical of this condition are recorded on the phonocardiogram.

11.8a–d Dextrocardia

There are always two atrial chambers, which show four possible arrangements. The normal right–left arrangement (solitus) may be mirror-imaged (inversus). Alternatively, two morphologically right or two morphologically left atria may be present (iso morphism). In general, the atrial situs maybe inferred from the visceral situs. Thus, if the chest radiograph shows a left-sided air bubble, the atrial situs is likely to be solitus. If the chest radiograph shows a right-sided air bubble, the atrial situs is likely to be inversus. The AV connection may be concordant or discordant depending on whether the atria are connected to their morphologically appropriate ventricle.

11.8a Dextrocardia: ECG. Note the P wave inversion and the deep S wave in standard lead 1.

With the V leads arranged around the left side of the chest (the normal arrangement) there is no progression of R wave.

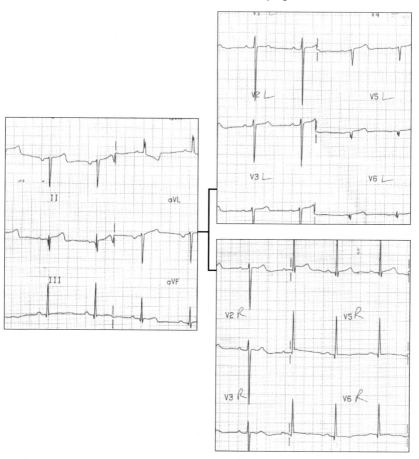

However, with the V leads arranged around the right side of the chest, the normal R wave progression is seen.

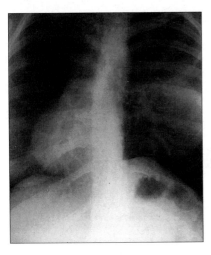

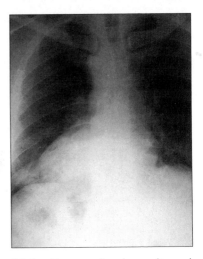

11.8b Dextrocardia: chest radiograph (situs solitus). Note that the heart is in the right side of the chest but the gastric air bubble is in the normal left-sided position.

11.8c Dextrocardia: chest radiograph (situs inversus). Here, dextrocardia is associated with a right-sided gastric air bubble indicating situs inversus.

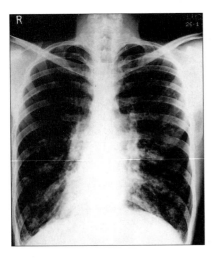

11.8d Kartagener's syndrome. The syndrome consists of the triad of sinusitis, bronchiectasis and situs inversus with dextrocardia. The disorder is inherited as an autosomal recessive trait. The chest radiograph shows dextrocardia and lung field abnormalities consistent with bronchiectasis.

11.9a and b   Ebstein's anomaly

Ebstein's anomaly is characterized by displacement of the septal attachment of the tricuspid valve towards the cardiac apex, increasing the size of the right atrium at the expense of the ventricle. Tricuspid regurgitation invariably occurs and 50% of patients have an ASD. Shunting may be from right to left because RA pressure is elevated, producing cyanosis, particularly in the newborn. As pulmonary resistance falls after birth, however, shunting decreases and cyanosis often disappears. Presentation may be at birth with heart failure and cyanosis but many patients develop symptoms insidiously over several years as RV function deteriorates.

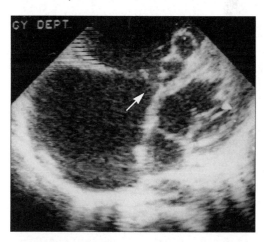

11.9a   Ebstein's anomaly: 2–D echocardiogram (four-chamber view). The septal attachment of the tricuspid valve (arrowed) is displaced towards the apex. Note the massive RA dilatation.

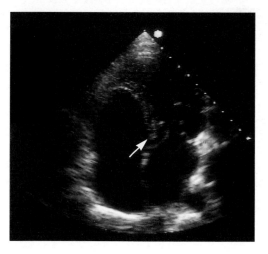

11.9b   Ebstein's anomaly: 2-D echocardiogram (four-chamber view). Again, the septal attachment of the tricuspid valve (arrowed) is displaced towards the apex causing massive dilatation of the right atrium.

11.10a and b Holt–Oram syndrome

About 25% of patients with defects of the radial side of the forearm and hands have congenital heart disease (usually ASD or VSD). This is probably because differentiation of the arm and the heart, particularly cardiac septation, both begin during the 4th week of gestation and are subject, therefore, to teratogenesis during this period.

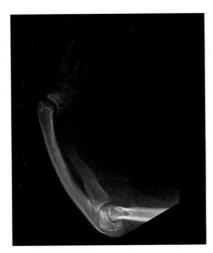

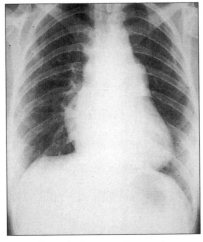

11.10a Holt–Oram syndrome: radiograph of forearm. Note the deformity of the radius in this patient.

11.10b Holt–Oram syndrome: chest radiograph. The patient had an ASD. Note the prominent main pulminary artery and the plethoric lung fields.

11.11a and b Cor triatriatum

In this uncommon anomaly a membrane representing the remnant of the common pulmonary vein separates the left atrium into two compartments. The proximal chamber receives the pulmonary veins whereas the distal chamber is related to the mitral valve and left atrial appendage. The membrane obstructs flow and presentation is usually in childhood with symptoms of pulmonary hypertension and chronic chest infections.

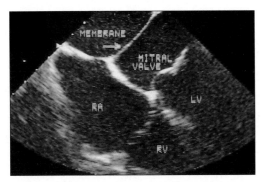

11.11a Cor triatriatum: transosopheageal echocardiogram. The membrane in the left atrium is clearly visible.

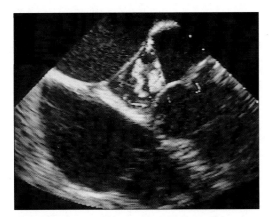

11.11b Cor triatriatum: transoesophageal echocardiogram with colour Doppler. This colour flow study shows flow across the central part of the membrane.

12.

Cardiac Tumours

12.1a–g Intracardiac thrombus

Thrombus is the most common cause of an intracardiac mass requiring differentiation from other tumours. Thrombus in the left side of the heart predisposes to systemic embolism whereas thrombus in the right side of the heart predisposes to pulmonary embolism.

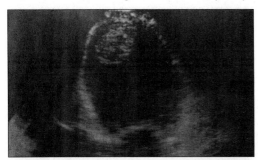

12.1a Intracardiac thrombus: 2-D echocardiogram. There is a large filling defect at the apex of the left ventricle caused by thrombus. The patient had recently had an extensive antero-apical infarct.

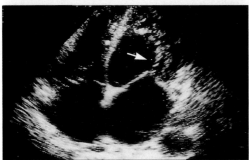

12.1b Intracardiac thrombus: 2-D echocardiogram. In this example, thrombus (arrowed) is layered over the apical and lateral walls of the left ventricle in a patient with long-standing coronary heart disease.

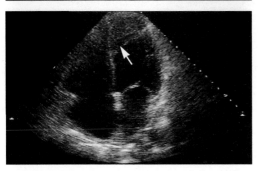

12.1c Intracardiac thrombus: 2-D echocardiogram. Here, layered thrombus (arrowed) is shown at the cardiac apex in relation to a previous myocardial infarct.

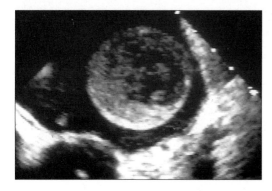

12.1d Intracardiac thrombus: transoesophageal echocardiogram. A large, organised ball thrombus is shown lying within the left atrial cavity.

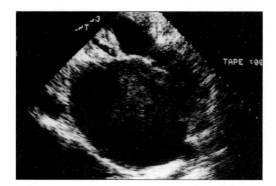

12.1e Spontaneous intracardiac echo-contrast: 2-D echocardiogram. The left atrium is massively dilated. Note the spontaneous echo-contrast caused by stasis of blood within the dilated chamber. The patient is clearly at high risk of developing an LA thrombus and requires anticoagulation therapy.

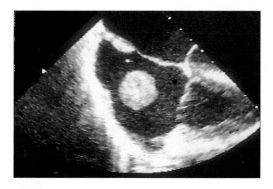

12.1f Intracardiac thrombus: transoesophageal echocardiogram. The patient was a transplant recipient and had developed a thrombotic mass in the right atrium in relation to the suture line.

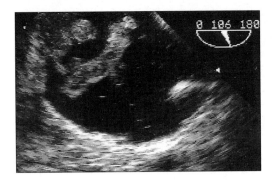

12.1g Intracardiac thrombus: transoesophageal echocardiogram. A serpiginous thrombotic mass is seen lying free in the right atrial cavity in this patient who had experienced massive pulmonary embolism caused by migration of thrombus from the ilio-femoral veins.

12.2a–f Benign cardiac tumours

Primary cardiac tumours are rare and the histologically benign myxoma accounts for at least one-half of all cases. In most patients, myxomas arise in the left atrium and are attached to the septum with prolapse into the mitral valve orifice during diastole. This impedes diastolic filling of the left ventricle and produces symptoms similar to mitral stenosis.

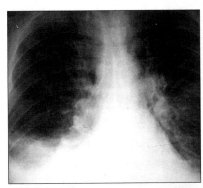

12.2a LA myxoma: chest radiograph. The heart is not enlarged but there is severe pulmonary oedema without clear signs of LA dilatation. The patient had an LA myxoma confirmed by echocardiography.

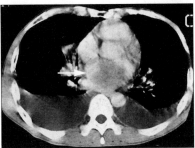

12.2b LA myxoma: CT scan. The posteriorly located left atrium is dilated and contains a filling defect (arrowed). Note the bilateral pleural effusions lying posteriorly in the chest.

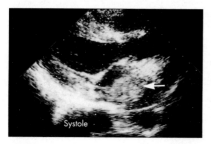
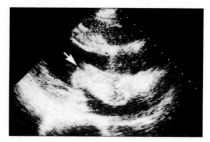

12.2c LA myxoma: 2-D echocardiogram (long axis view). During diastole, the tumour (arrowed) prolapses through the mitral valve, obstructing LV filling.

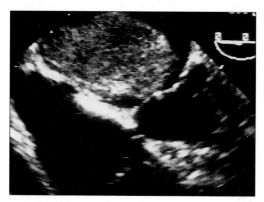

12.2d LA myxoma: transoesophageal echocardiogram. There is a large myxoma in the left atrium attached to the inter-atrial septum.

12.2e LA myxoma: MRI scan.

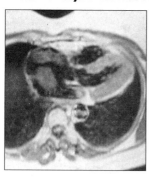
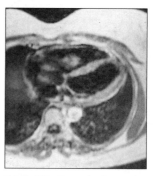

12.2e(i) Systolic frame. A lobulated myxoma is clearly seen within the left atrium.

12.2e(ii) Diastolic frame during diastole one lobe prolapses through the mitral valve

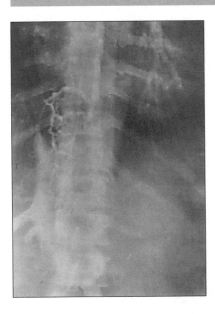

12.2f Intracardiac leiomyoma: inferior vena-cavagram. This is a rare, histologically benign tumour. It derives from the vascular bed of the uterus and may grow along the uterine veins into the inferior vena cava and progress upwards towards the right atrium. This patient presented with evidence of tricuspid valve obstruction. Note the large filling defect in the inferior vena cava and the prominent collateral veins.

12.3a–e Malignant cardiac tumours

Primary malignant disease of the heart is rare, sarcomas accounting for all cases. Much more common is metastatic disease, usually originating from the breast or lung.

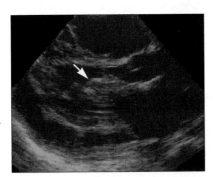
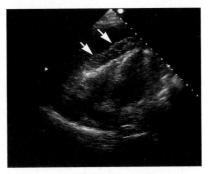

12.3a Cardiac fibrosarcoma: 2-D echocardiogram (long axis view). A large tumour (arrowed) is adherent to the anterior leaflet of the mitral valve. Pericardial seeding has resulted in pericardial effusion.

12.3b Metastatic tumour: 2-D echocardiogram (apical view). Note the tumour (arrowed) layered along the free wall of the right ventricle and encroaching on the cardiac apex. This has resulted in a large pericardial effusion.

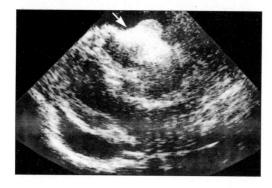

12.3c Cardiac fibrosarcoma: 2-D echocardiogram (long axis view). A large mass is apparent (arrowed) attached to the free wall of the right ventricle, resulting in pericardial effusion.

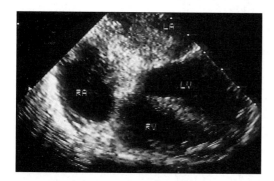

12.3d Cardiac lymphoma: transoesophageal echocardiogram. There is a large diffuse mass involving the interatrial septum and encroaching on the left atrial cavity. The patient had a mediastinal lymphoma which had invaded the heart.

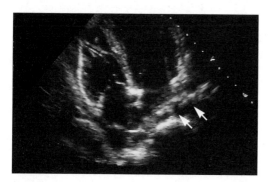

12.3e Extracardiac lymphoma: 2-D echocardiogram (four-chamber view). The patient had a mediastinal lymphoma. Note how the left atrium is distorted (arrows) because of compression by the tumour mass.

13.

Pulmonary Heart Disease

13.1a–h Acute pulmonary embolism

Acute pulmonary embolism is usually a complication of deep venous thrombosis involving the ilio-femoral veins. Its severity is determined by the extent of pulmonary vascular obstruction but only when it exceeds 50% (massive embolism) does pulmonary resistance rise sufficiently to cause right ventricular failure. Minor embolism is often clinically silent, occasionally causing pleurisy and haemoptysis. Massive embolism presents with abrupt onset dyspnoea and chest pain; shock and sudden death may occur. Treatment is with heparin and oxygen; in severe cases, thrombolytic therapy or even embolectomy may be necessary.

Risk factors for deep venous thrombosis
Immobility Particularly after hip and abdominal surgery
Venous stasis in legs Varicose veins, vena cava compression (e.g. gravid uterus), bony fractures of legs
Heart disease Myocardial infarction, heart failure
Endocrine/metabolic factors Diabetes, obesity, contraceptive pill, postpartum period
Malignant disease Particularly pancreatic and bronchial carcinoma
Miscellaneous Polycythaemia, Behçet's disease

13.1a Risk factors for deep venous thrombosis. The immobility that follows major surgery is undoubtedly the major risk for deep venous thrombosis. Heparin prophylaxis is of proven benefit and should be offered to patients at risk.

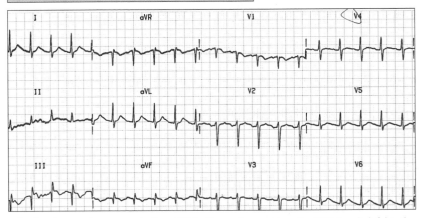

13.1b Acute pulmonary embolism: ECG. Generally speaking, the ECG is unhelpful in the diagnosis of pulmonary embolism. However, in massive pulmonary embolism, tachycardia and signs of acute right heart strain (S1, Q3, T3) may be evident, as in this example.

13.1c(i) and (ii) Acute pulmonary embolism: ventilation–perfusion isotope lung scan.

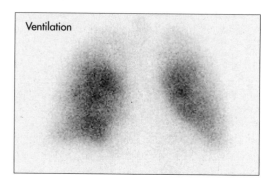

Ventilation

13.1c(i) In pulmonary embolism, alveolar ventilation remains normal and the ventilation scan shows homogeneous distribution of isotope.

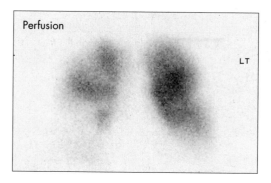

Perfusion

LT

13.1c(ii) Blood flow to those parts of the lungs subtended by the obstructed vessel (or vessels), however, is impaired and the perfusion scan shows regional defects. The demonstration of ventilation–perfusion 'mismatch' is highly specific for pulmonary embolism.

13.1d (i) and (ii) Acute pulmonary embolism: 2-D echocardiogram (four-chamber view).

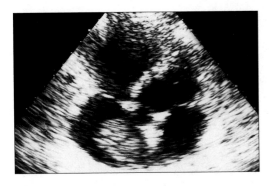

13.1d (i) Systolic frame. A large thrombotic mass is visible in the right atrium. This is a thrombus that has migrated from the ilio-femoral veins in a patient with massive pulmonary embolism.

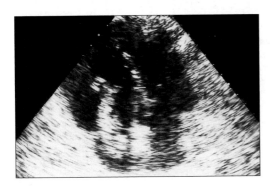

13.1d (ii) Diastolic frame. Note the thrombolic mass prolapses through the tricuspid valvein diastole. Migration into the pulmonary artery is inevitable.

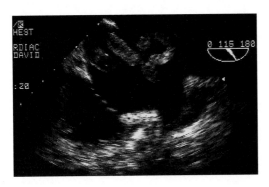

13.1e Acute pulmonary embolism: transoesophageal echocardiogram. At least two, perhaps three, sausage-shaped masses are visible in the right ventricle. These are thrombi that have migrated from the ilio-femoral veins in a patient with massive pulmonary embolism.

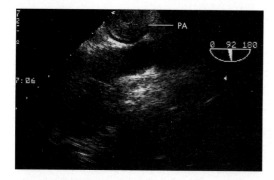

13.1f Acute pulmonary embolism: transoesophageal echocardiogram. In this view, the pulmonary artery (PA) is lying in close relation to the transducer with the aorta in front. Note how the pulmonary artery is almost completely obliterated by thrombus in this patient with massive pulmonary embolism.

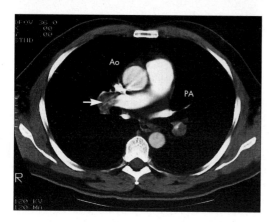

13.1g Acute pulmonary embolism: CT scan. The contrast-enhanced pulmonary artery (PA) is seen behind the aorta (Ao). The contrast column in the pulmonary artery terminates abruptly because of a large thrombotic mass (arrowed) occluding its lumen.

13.1h Acute pulmonary embolism: angiography. Selective left and right pulmonary angiograms are shown.

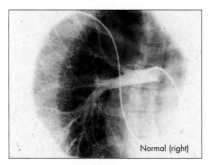 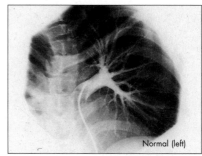

13.1h(i) This normal study shows homogeneous distribution of contrast throughout both lung fields.

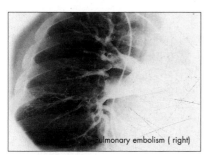 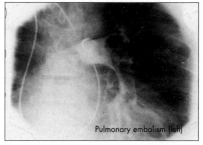

13.1h(ii) Massive pulmonary embolism: note the large filling defect in the proximal part of the left pulmonary artery effectively restricting flow to the lower zone of the left lung. Filling defects are also seen in the major branches of the right pulmonary artery.

13.2a–c Chronic pulmonary embolism

Chronic pulmonary embolism usually remains clinically silent until repeated embolic episodes with progressive obliteration of the vascular bed cause advanced pulmonary hypertension. Treatment with long term warfarin is directed at preventing further embolism but prognosis is poor.

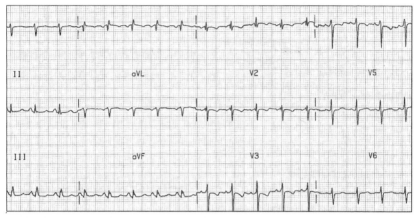

13.2a Chronic pulmonary embolism: ECG. Note the P pulmonale, right axis deviation and the dominant R wave in lead V1. These are typical features of pulmonary hypertension.

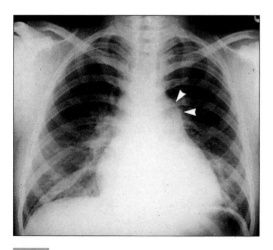

13.2b Chronic pulmonary embolism: chest radiograph. Long-standing pulmonary hypertension has produced cardiac enlargement with dilatation of the main pulmonary artery (arrowed).

13.2c(i) and (ii)   Chronic pulmonary embolism: selective pulmonary angiography. Contrast has been hand-injected through a balloon-tipped catheter wedged in a branch of the pulmonary artery.

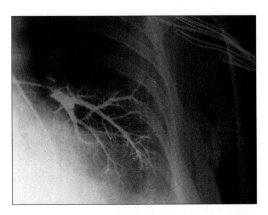

13.2c(i) Normal study. Note the fine recticular pattern of the pulmonary arterial tree.

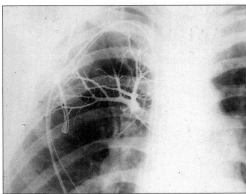

13.2c(ii) Pulmonary embolism. Note the fine recticular pattern is lost in this patient with severe pulmonary hyper–tension.

13.3a–e Primary pulmonary hypertension

This is an uncommon disorder, usually affecting young women. Obliterative pulmonary arteriolar disease of unknown cause results in progressive pulmonary hypertension and right ventricular failure. Prognosis is poor and heart and lung transplantation is the only effective treatment.

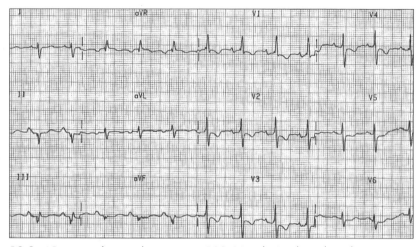

13.3a   Primary pulmonary hypertension: ECG. Note the P pulmonale, right axis deviation and prominent R wave in lead V1. Similar changes are seen in 13.2a (chronic pulmonary embolism) and reflect the severe pulmonary hypertension characteristic of both conditions.

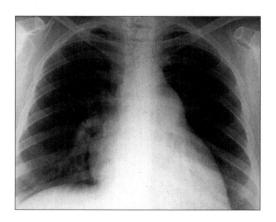

13.3b   Primary pulmonary hypertension: chest radiograph. Note the cardiac enlargement, the marked dilatation of the proximal pulmonary arteries and the relatively oligaemic lung fileds.

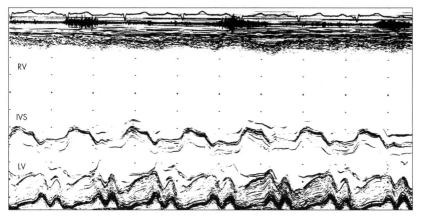

13.3c Primary pulmonary hypertension: M-mode echocardiogram. There is massive dilatation of the right ventricle. LV cavity dimensions are normal but note the paradoxical movement of the interventricular septum which moves inward during diastole (arrowed). RV dilatation of this severity is a nonspecific feature of long standing pulmonary hypertension.

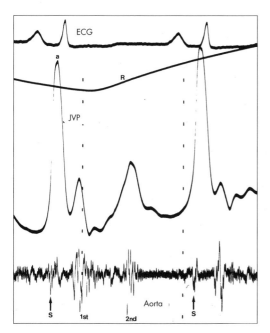

13.3d Primary pulmoanry hypertension: venous pulse recording. Note the giant 'a' wave and the fourth heart sound (S), both reflecting the vigorous atrial systole required to fill the hypertropied right ventricle.

References

Figure 3.13   From: Mock M.B. Ringqvist I, Fisher LD, *et al*. Survival of medically treated patients in the Coronary Artery Study (CASS) registry. Circulation 1982, **66**:562–8.

Figure 3.16a   Data from Newham General Hospital CCU database. Reproduced by permission of Dr Timmis.

Figure 3.20b and c   Data from Timmis AD, Griffin B, Nelson DJ, Sowton E. The effects of early coronary patency on the evolution of myocardial infarction: a prospective arteriographic study. *Br Heart J*, **58**:345–51.

Figure 3.20d   Ranjadayalan, UmachandranV, Timmis AD. The effects of thrombolytic therapy on temperature responses to acute myocardial infarction. *C A D* 1991, **2**: 907–12.

Figure 3.26a   Stevenson R, Ranjadayalan K, Wilkinson P, Roberts R, Timmis AD. Short- and -long term prognosis of acute myocardial infarction since introduction of thrombolysis. *Br Med J* 1993, **307**: 349–53.

Figure 3.26b   Laji K, Wilkinson P, Ranjadayalan K, Timmis AD. Prognosis in acute myocardial infarction: comparison of patients with diagnostic and nondiagnostic electrocardiograms. *Am Heart J* 1995, **130**: 705–10.

Figure 3.26c   Stevenson R, UmachanadranV, Ranjadayalan K, Marchant B, Timmis AD. Reassessment of treadmill stress testing for risk stratification in patients with acute myocardial infarction treated by thrombolysis. *Br Heart J* 1993, **70**:415–20.

Figure 3.26d   The Multicenter Postinfarction Research Group. Risk stratification and survival after myocardial infarction. *N Engl J Med* 1983, 331–6.

Figure 4.13b   Cohn JN, Archibald DG, Ziesche S, *et al*. Effect of vasodilator therapy on mortality in chronic congestive heart failure: results of a Veterans Administration Cooperative Study. *N Engl J Med* 1986, **314**: 1547–52.

Figure 4.14a   CONSENSUS Trial Study Group. Effects of enalapril on mortality in severe congestive heart failure results of the Cooperative North Scandinavian enalapril Survival Study (CONSENSUS). *N Engl J Med* 1987, **316**: 1429–35.

Figure 4.15a   The SOLVD Investigators. Effect of enalapril on survival in patients with reduced left ventricular ejection fractions and congestive heart failure. *N Engl J Med* 1991, **325**: 293–302.

Figure 4.15c   The SOLVD Investigators. Effect of enalapril on mortality and development of heart failure in asymptomatic patients with reduced left ventricular ejection fractions. *N Engl Med* 1992, **327**: 685–91.

Figure 4.16   Packer M, Carver JR, Rodeheffer RJ, *et al*. For the PROMISE Study Group. Effect of oral milrinone on mortality in severe chronic heart failure. *N Engl J Med* 1991, **325**: 1468 –75.

Index